THE F

The Fasting Key

How You Can Unlock Doors to Spiritual Blessing

Mark Nysewander

Vine Books
Servant Publications
Ann Arbor, Michigan

Vine Books is an imprint of Servant Publications especially designed to serve evangelical Christians.

Servant Publications – Mission Statement
We are dedicated to publishing books that spread the gospel of Jesus Christ, help Christians to live in accordance with that gospel, promote renewal in the church, and bear witness to Christian unity.

Servant Publications
P.O. Box 8617
Ann Arbor, MI 48107
www.servantpub.com

Cover design by CCD, www.ccdgroup.co.uk

04 05 06 07 10 9 8 7 6 5 4 3 2 1

Printed in the United States of America

ISBN 1-56955-363-7

To my wife, Kathy,
who has prayed, fasted and believed with me
through both the good and the difficult times,
and to our three children,
Jenny, Dwight and John Mark,
sources of joy and encouragement.

Contents

Foreword

Anyone who is watching the landscape of Christianity is noticing the resurgence of prayer, fasting and worship in the Body of Christ. The Holy Spirit is awakening the Church to the reality of radical Christianity by restoring the simple, ancient paths which lead to fervent love and whole-hearted abandonment to Jesus. Fasting is a great gift in the grace of God that enlarges our capacity to receive more of Jesus. *The Fasting Key* describes how, through the seemingly weak means of fasting, God is strategically awakening the Bride of Christ to the beautiful presence and unrivaled power of her Bridegroom King, Christ Jesus.

Mike Bickle
International House of Prayer of Kansas City

Introduction

On Assignment from God

Steve was a heroin-addicted hippie living in a trailer park outside Sydney. Sitting on the steps of his trailer he noticed an unfamiliar car drive into the grounds. Out jumped an elderly man and his wife. The old man shouted, "Praise the Lord!" Then the couple approached Steve and gave a description of a girl they were trying to find. They wanted to share some food and clothes with her. Recognizing the description, Steve pointed to where the girl lived. Steve asked the man if he worked with the government welfare agency. The man smiled and said he didn't. He then explained that he had been fasting and praying. God had given him a vision of the girl they were now looking for and had shown him the trailer park where she lived. He had never before met her or been to the trailer park. The couple had driven hundreds of miles in obedience to the vision that came through the old man's fast.

That night the couple, Henry and Mural Gallus, had a little cookout and invited Steve and his friends to come and eat with them. Walking up, Steve noticed off in the distance that it was raining to the north, south, east and west but it wasn't raining where they were. Steve asked Henry what was going on. He explained that he had asked the Lord to hold off the rain for the cookout and gospel presentation. He wanted to share with Steve and his friends about Jesus. Before the night was over Steve was kneeling on his kitchen floor crying out to Jesus for the forgiveness of his sins. Weeping on the floor beside him was Henry.

Fasting comes to my life

Ten years later I met Steve when he, his wife and daughters came to Wilmore, Kentucky, where Steve attended Asbury Seminary. Steve would share stories of his old friend and how Henry had lived a lifestyle of fasting until he died at age seventy-seven. Steve possessed Henry's diaries that stretched over fifty years of Christian life. They included many references to long periods of fasting. The diaries also told of extraordinary experiences in answer to his prayer and fasting.

As I heard Steve tell of Henry's exploits for the Lord all over Australia, I was drawn more and more into fasting. Steve loaned me some tapes of Henry's teachings. I was shocked at the number of references throughout the Bible to fasting. This was not some biblical side issue. It was central to spiritual life. I soon began to see fasting throughout church history and in the lives of men and women of God. Since those days when I first met Steve, fasting has become an essential part of my walk with the Lord. It continues to amaze me that I lived for so long without this key which unlocks so many blessings.

Revivals everywhere

I am indebted to a man on the other side of the earth whom I never met: Henry Gallus. His anointing for fasting has somehow drawn me into fasting. I write this book believing that you too will discover this lost key to incredible kingdom resources. May God raise up an army of fasting warriors that will unlock the doors to a world-wide revival. Henry Gallus was convinced the fasting key could open up such a blessing. He once wrote, "If the millions of Christians took fasting as seriously as they took praying and giving, in a matter of weeks a wave of righteousness would sweep over this world, which would be felt and recorded by revivals everywhere."[1]

I pray you will be one of those millions who will ignite a chain reaction of global revivals through your fasting.

To God be the Glory

Mark Nysewander

1. Henry Gallus, *Sanctify A Fast* (Blenheim: Back to the Bible Pub., 1954) p. 19

Chapter 1

The Lost Key

"On that day they will fast."
(Mark 2:20)

Lost and Forgotten

I carry a key ring with a set of keys, each of which opens a different door in our church. Unfortunately the western Church has lost an important key. It unlocks many doors to resources that are essential for you and me as believers. Isaiah 58 speaks of this lost key and the kingdom resources it opens to us. Here are some of the resources mentioned: protection, revelation, provision, revival, God's presence, deliverance and much more. Not only have you and I lost this key but it has been so long since we used it we have even forgotten about its existence. Think what it would be like if you never prayed. Now take it a step further. What would it be like if you not only never prayed, but completely forgot about the existence of prayer?

In the sixth chapter of Matthew's Gospel, Jesus talks about three essential keys you should use if you are to live a kingdom life. One of these keys is prayer and the other key is giving. Both of these you frequently use. But the third key that opens up a storehouse of kingdom resources is not just a lost key. It is a forgotten key. Most believers never think of it. A few use it rarely. This key has been misplaced because of several misunderstandings. Each misunderstanding deceives us into believing that this key is useless, dangerous or foolish. The lost key I am referring to is fasting. It is my prayer that God will give you discernment to see any misunderstanding that keeps you from using the fasting key.

A relic from the past

One popular misunderstanding claims that fasting is no more than a leftover from an old religious practice. It therefore holds no value for us today. Fasting is seen as a primitive religious ritual that some folks around the world use but which has nothing to do with our progressive church life. We have moved beyond all that.

Recently I heard about a group of visitors from the United States checking out Pastor David Cho's church in Korea. It is the largest church in the world. They asked the Korean believers, "What is the secret of this church's growth?" The Koreans answered that it was fasting and prayer. But the Americans demanded, "Yes, but besides that what are you doing to make this church grow?" We just don't believe that fasting is an essential key to release the resources of the kingdom. We refuse to examine it. For many of us anything else besides fasting will do.

Abstinence is not fasting

The second misunderstanding about fasting claims that all abstinence is fasting. If you abstain from sex, from TV, from chocolate or football then that is a fast. No! That is abstinence but it is not a fast. It has its own value in our spiritual life but don't call it a fast. In the Old

Testament the word fasting simply means, "to cover your mouth." In the New Testament it means, "not to eat." So biblical fasting is to do without food.

The other extreme of this misunderstanding about fasting states that anytime you do without food, it is a fast. That too is wrong. Not all absence of food is biblical fasting. If you think you are fasting because you are on a diet, anorexic, fasting for health reasons, or joining a hunger strike you are mistaken. None of these are the fasting you find in the Scriptures. Simply to abstain from food is not a biblical fast.

So what is the lost key? Fasting is to quit eating for an agreed period of time. The agreement is between you and the Lord or you and other believers. You do it for the glory of God. That is the important part. It is not a political or even religious statement. It is not to lose weight. It is not even to clean out your system of toxins. Some of these things will happen in a fast. But you only fast to bring glory to God in your life, church and community.

When you fast from food, continue to drink water, unless it is an extreme fast – which is a waterless fast. If it is an extreme fast you should never go beyond three days without water. A supernatural fast is when someone goes longer than three days without water and food. Moses completed such a fast. He did it twice for forty days each time (Deuteronomy 9:9, 18). It was a miracle and should never be tried by human decision and strength.

A command or an option

There is also a misunderstanding about the necessity of fasting. To many people fasting is seen as a heavy, legalistic command that holds no life or joy. When Jesus was here on this earth He refused to make fasting a law that had to be obeyed. In Mark 2:18–20 Jesus was asked why He and His disciples didn't fast like the other spiritual groups. He said it wasn't time to fast. It was time to feast. Fasting is not some law to obey at the expense of crushing times of celebration and joy. To Jesus it was just as much a sin to fast on a feast day as to feast on a fast day. If fasting becomes a heavy legalism it is not the fasting of the Scriptures. Most believers, on the other hand, often see fasting as an option for Christians. It is viewed on the same level as foot washing or some other optional experience in the Bible. Could fasting be so important that it is more than an option?

John Wesley, the great revivalist of England, did not see fasting as an option. He said, "The man that never fasts is no more on the way to heaven than the man who never prays."[1] Wesley wasn't proposing that fasting was the means of our salvation. He was saying it is the fruit of salvation, which refers to Jesus' teaching from the Sermon on the Mount. In that great message notice Jesus doesn't say, "If you fast," as though you had an option. He says, *"When you fast"* (Matthew 6:16). To Jesus, fasting is an expected practice, as much as praying and giving. There is no option.

Fasting is a passion

If fasting is not a command or an option, what is it? Jesus proclaims,

> *"The time will come, when the bridegroom will be taken from them, and on that day they will fast."*
>
> (Mark 2:20)

We now live in that day. Jesus is taken away physically and sits in heaven at the right hand of the Father. Notice He doesn't suggest that fasting is an option for He says in this present time *"they will fast."* The disciples of Jesus now fast because of a fiery love for their absent bridegroom. Fasting is a means of communing with your absent bridegroom. When Jesus was physically present on earth fasting wasn't necessary for fellowship with Him. Now you fast to know Him.

Because you are born again, Jesus was convinced, sooner or later, that the Spirit of God would lead you into periods of fasting. Not because you have to do it or even because fasting is a neat option to try. You fast out of your passion for Jesus who is your all in all.[2]

Fasting brings results

There is also a misunderstanding about the results of fasting. Fasting brings incredible resources of the kingdom into your life. But the enemy pushes the misunderstanding that there is no benefit in a fast. After all, what does not eating have to do with your spiritual life? Be clear about this. When you fast there are results! Jesus promised that those who engage in secret fasting would be openly rewarded (Matthew 6:18). Expect the Lord to add new kingdom resources to your life as you fast.

Another misunderstanding is to presume the result will always be exactly and immediately what you want. Results will come but they are not always immediate or predictable. At times, results are gradual and tend to diversify as you give yourself more and more to fasting. God responds to your fast. Maybe not in the timing and manner you originally thought He would. But He openly rewards you. Remember, these kingdom resources often come through a lifestyle of fasting instead of a one-time fast.

Showers of blessing

Get ready because there will be results. Fasting is the key

that unlocks the doors to the incredible resources of the kingdom. Sadhu Sundar Singh, a traveling teacher and preacher in India, discovered this truth. He once shared how a forty-day fast opened the door to a new consciousness of the Lord Jesus. He explained that in India there are long periods of rainless heat. When the first rain comes, the heat rises, mixes with the dust and forms a hot mist. It creates a sense of suffocation. But after subsequent showers there is no more hot mist or feeling of suffocation. The Sadhu shared that after the first shower of grace, which was his conversion, he felt the perplexities and suffocating mist of the external world. Then he fasted. It was like the subsequent showers of blessings. He came into a greater consciousness of spiritual things. He discovered a deeper experience of the Lord Jesus.[3]

Fasting is not an option, nor is it some kind of legal command. It is a means of grace for spiritual blessing. Give the Spirit opportunity to lead you into fasting. Discover this long lost key that will open up new experiences of the Lord's presence and grace. As the Sadhu discovered, fasting leads to a fuller communion with your Lord Jesus Christ. After all He is your greatest blessing.

Notes

1. John Wesley, *Sermons on Several Occasions*, (London: Wesleyan Conference Office, 1868) Vol 3, Sermon 116, Section 14, p. 276
2. Arthur Wallis, *God's Chosen Fast* (Pennsylvania: Christian Literature Crusade, 1968) p. 23
3. B.H. Steeter, *The Message of Sadhu Sundar Singh* (New York: The Macmillan Company, 1921) p. 66

Chapter 2

The Useless Key

"You cannot fast as you do today and expect your voice to be heard on high."
(Isaiah 58:4b)

A Bad Copy

Once I had a key made for a door and it looked just like the original key. But when I tried to use the new key it didn't work. There was a small defect that kept the key from functioning correctly. The copied key was not much different from the original key. They looked the same but there was enough difference to make the copied key useless. The door would not open.

Fasting is the lost key to kingdom living. But there is also a bad key out there. It looks just like true fasting but it has a defect that keeps it from opening up all the resources of the kingdom. A bad fast is done out of a wrong motive. That is what makes it defective. Of the seventy-one fasts or references to fasting in the Bible, seven of them have to do with a bad fast. These are useless keys that will not open the doors of heaven's warehouse. Isaiah 58 describes the characteristics of a bad fast. When I first saw these characteristics, I presumed the way to avoid a bad fast was not to fast at all. But the scripture is not suggesting that we avoid fasting. It is simply showing us the kind of fasting we should avoid. What are the defective motives that make fasting useless?

Fasting for image

Don't fast to look religious. Isaiah 58:2 says of those who do a bad fast, *"they seem eager to know my ways"* and *"they ... seem eager for God to come near them."* These people were acting as if they wanted God when in fact they didn't. Fasting was just a way to make a good religious impression. In other words, a bad fast is when you fast to look good to others and to God. You really don't want God. You just want to look like you want God.

In Zechariah 7:5 God asks,

> *"When you fasted and mourned in the fifth and seventh months for the past seventy years, was it really for me that you fasted?"*

As you can see, the Jews had fasted over a seventy-year period. God, however, wanted to know who was the object of their fast. If it's not for God, who else can you fast for?

Jesus answers this question in Luke 18:9–14. Here He tells the story of a very religious man, a Pharisee, who fasted and prayed regularly. In verse 11 Jesus says that the Pharisee *"prayed about himself."* Do you understand? He fasted and prayed to make himself look good and religious. He wanted to impress both God and others. He wasn't fasting for God. He was fasting for his religious image. When you fast and it's not for God, you are fasting for yourself. As Jesus speaks of fasting in the Sermon on the Mount He warns us about fasting to impress people with our religion (Matthew 6:16–18). If that is your motive then your only reward will be a bunch of impressed people. You will not know the kingdom resources that come from God.

One of the early church fathers, St. Mark the Ascetic, lived about four hundred years after Jesus spoke about fasting in the Sermon on the Mount. He too warned, "Fasting while of value in itself, is not something to boast of in front of God."[1] It is a bad fast when you use fasting as a way to boast of your religiousness. That is a useless key that only opens up an inflated ego!

On the other hand, don't fall into a legalistic secrecy about fasting. I have known people who believe that telling anyone they are fasting is boasting. In order to keep their fasting a secret, they will lie about why they are not eating. Jesus is not asking you to lie or deceive your friends and family. He is simply warning you not to boast. Whenever necessary explain that you are fasting. Do it humbly, without boasting in front of God or others. After all, Jesus must have told someone about His forty-day fast or it would not be recorded in the Bible.

Fasting as a merit badge

A bad fast is when you fast not just to look religious but to be religious. Some folks see fasting as a way to merit God's response because of their goodness through fasting. In Isaiah 58:3 the people are upset with God because He hasn't responded to them though they have been religious.

> *" 'Why have we fasted,' they say,*
> *'and you have not seen it?*
> *Why have we humbled ourselves,*
> *and you have not noticed?' "*

But these people are not interested in holiness or in knowing God. They fast to be religious. Do you see fasting as a religious way of acting so God will give you what you want? If so, you have a wrong motive that will cause your fasting to be a useless key. It will not open the doors of the kingdom of God. It will open wide the doors of religion.

Fasting is not some kind of goodness that makes God respond to your desires. When David fasted for God to stop the judgment against his family because of his sins, God didn't respond to his fasting (2 Samuel 12:15–23). He didn't have to! Fasting doesn't guarantee that God has to do what you want.

John Wesley warned his people of this bad fasting when he said,

> "Let us beware of fancying we merit anything of God by our fasting."[2]

And centuries earlier St. Makarios, a church father, writes,

> "Indeed, the cardinal rule of the Christian life is not to put one's trust in acts of righteousness even if one practices all of them, or to imagine that one has done anything great."[3]

That is the point. You haven't done anything great. You haven't merited anything of God by your fasting. Fasting is not a religious act that impresses God and causes Him to respond to your desires. It's fine to fast for a particular answer to your prayer or a need in your life. Believe in the power of God that comes through fasting. But never assume fasting is a goodness that forces God to give you what you want. Fasting is simply a way to increase your faith and press into the presence of God. Put your faith in God, not in fasting.

Fasting to feed a religious spirit

Fasting is also useless when you do it out of a religious spirit. Isaiah 58:3–4 describes a people who fast even as they sin. That is the work of a religious spirit. The Lord reveals,

> *"Yet on the day of your fasting, you do as you please*
> *and exploit all your workers.*
> *Your fasting ends in quarreling and strife,*
> *and in striking each other with wicked fists."*

The Lord has a strong rebuke. He warns,

> *"You cannot fast as you do today*
> *and expect your voice to be heard on high."*

It is useless fasting.

It is not only useless. It is dangerous. This kind of fasting feeds a religious spirit. Soon you are taking the sacred gifts of God's grace and using them to cover your rebellion against God. You move from continuing in sin as you fast, to concealing your sin with a fast. To use fasting this way is to be in the company of Jezebel. She orders a national day of fasting to help conceal her plot to murder Naboth and take his vineyard. She declares a fast for the sole purpose of providing a religious cover for her sinful act (1 Kings 21:9–14). You can guard against this religious spirit by fasting with repentance before the Lord. David declares in Psalm 51:16–17 that God does not delight in sacrifice or burnt offerings but in a broken spirit and a contrite heart. Fasting is a sacrifice because you are not eating food. But God does not delight in the sacrifice of fasting by itself. You must also turn away from sin and repent. Otherwise it is a useless sacrifice that can be the inspiration of a religious spirit.

A form of godliness

Finally, a fast is useless when it is no more than a religious ritual. In Isaiah 58:5 God questions the ritual fasting of His people. He says,

> *"Is this the kind of fast I have chosen,*
> *only a day for a man to humble himself?*
> *Is it only for bowing one's head like a reed*
> *and for lying on sackcloth and ashes?*
> *Is this what you call a fast,*
> *a day acceptable to the LORD?"*

These people are only fulfilling a ritual, without any desire to engage God in the fast. It is a dead ritual and it is also a useless key. You can ritualize fasting so that you have the form of godliness but deny its power (2 Timothy 3:5). You deny the power of godliness because you don't have faith. Whenever you fast for the sake of fulfilling religious ritual you are out of grace and into dead religion. Do you want to avoid making your fast a religious ritual devoid of any spiritual content? Believe God to work through your fast. Fasting is not something you do for God. It is a means of grace, entered into by faith, where God can do something in and through you by His Son, Jesus Christ.

Grind off all religion

Growing up, I worked at a store where I made keys. Sometimes customers would return saying the new key didn't work. I would examine the key and find some portion that needed to be ground off. When you enter into a fast make sure you grind off any religious portion. Fasting is not for religious looks to impress people, religious acts to get God's blessing, religious spirits to hide sin or religious ritual to fulfill duty. These imperfections will make fasting useless. Fast with faith. Believe God for greater measures of His presence and power in your life. Then watch the doors of blessings open.

Notes

1. G.E.H. Palmer, Philip Sherrard and Kallistos Ware – translators, *The Philokalia* (Boston: Faber and Faber, 1984), Vol. 3, p. 335
2. John Wesley, *Wesley's 52 Standard Sermons* (Salem: Schmul Pub. 1988) p. 285
3. G.E.H. Palmer, Philip Sherrard and Kallistos Ware – translators, *The Philokalia* (Boston: Faber and Faber, 1979), Vol. 1, p. 267

Chapter 3

The Master Key

"Is not this the kind of fast I have chosen . . ."
(Isaiah 58:6)

The Key That Works

There are two things you need to know about a master key. First, it opens every room in the building. Second, you only give a master key to someone you can trust. If you are handing over access into every locked room, give it to a person with integrity. In the last chapter you discovered the useless key of fasting. It will not open one single door to kingdom resources. It only opens up an inflated religious ego. That is a bad fast. But there is not only a bad fast. There is also a good fast. A good fast is more than a useful key. It is the master key.

Isaiah 58 describes the master key of fasting. It also describes the many doors in God's kingdom warehouse that can be opened by this key. But God only gives the master key to those who are responsible. A good fast is one that is done with a right motive. Here are the motives that are essential to a good fast.

Answering God's call

It is a good fast when you respond to God. In Isaiah 58:6 God asks, *"Is not this the kind of fast I have chosen?"* The implication is that a good fast is God initiated. The reason for your fast is to obey God's prompting. It is only done for His glory. Joel 1:14 declares, *"Declare a holy fast."* Set a fast apart for God. Fast because God has chosen it. Seek the Lord to see when you should fast, for how long and what should be the nature of your fast. Ask Him to show you the objectives for your fast.

Does this mean that fasting is always a spontaneous word from the Lord and should never be done on a routine basis? No. It could be that God's chosen fast for you is once a week, a certain meal each day, a corporate fast with your church or several days of fasting each month. In the same way as prayer comes in all shapes, sizes and seasons, so does fasting. Whether it is prayer, giving or fasting, you should seek the Lord's will and sanctify your expressions of righteousness by responding to His directions.

Maybe you believe God has never prompted you to fast. But have you asked Him? John Wesley told the early Methodists, "Fasting is only a way which God hath ordained, wherein we wait for his unmerited mercy."[1] It is only one way, but it is an ordained way and God will lead you to fast if you ask Him.

Satan fears fasting

It is a good fast when your motive is to defeat the enemy. Isaiah 58:6 says,

> *"Is not this the kind of fasting I have chosen:*
> *to loose the chains of injustice*
> *and untie the cords of the yoke,*

to set the oppressed free
and break every yoke."

There is no mention of Satan in this passage, but his fingerprints are everywhere. It speaks of cords, chains and yokes. These represent slavery, bondage and oppression. Whether Satan does his works of destruction through human or demonic instruments matters little. When you fast to loose the chains, untie the cords, break the yokes and set the captives free, it is a good fast. Jesus gives you a model for this kind of fasting. After Jesus received the baptism of John and the Holy Spirit, He fasted for forty days to confront Satan and his temptations (Matthew 4:1–2).

Like Jesus, your fasting can come against any bondage or temptation Satan is seeking to put on you. One church father, St. Hesychios, wrote,

> "He [Jesus] taught us, as feeble as we are, that we should fight against the demons with humility, fasting, prayer and watchfulness. For when, after His baptism, He went into the desert and the devil came up to Him as though He were merely a man, He began His spiritual warfare by fasting and won the battle by this means."[2]

Your fast cannot only free you but it can also free others from any bondage of the enemy. Joel 2:20 declares that God will drive the northern army far from the land because the people of God fast. Whether the army is a host of demonic spirits or a human army empowered by the demonic, fasting breaks its power!

Carlos Annacondia of Argentina has discovered that when he binds the enemy through weeks of fasting and prayer before he begins an evangelistic crusade, multitudes will be delivered and saved during the meeting.

Pablo Deiros reports that when Annacondia begins to rebuke the enemy "a powerful electricity goes through the people." A huge line of people files into the special deliverance tent every night of the crusade.[3]

Satan fears fasting. He fears it because fasting destroys his power. When you fast to break Satan's bondage in your life or in the lives of others, it's a good fast.

Fast with mercy

Your fast is good when you do it to help others. In Isaiah 58:7 God is speaking of the kind of fast He wants. He says,

> *"Is it not to share your food with the hungry*
> *and to provide the poor wanderer with shelter–*
> *when you see the naked, to clothe him,*
> *and not to turn away from your own flesh and blood?"*

A good fast that is committed to helping the needy can mean one of two things. It may mean your fasting is surrounded with acts of mercy. Fasting should come out of a lifestyle that seeks to help others. Feed the hungry, give shelter, clothe the naked and help your own family. In the Sermon on the Mount the Lord speaks of fasting within the context of praying and giving to those in need (Matthew 6:2, 5, 16). It is a good fast when other manifestations of righteousness accompany it. Giving to those in need is one such manifestation of righteousness.

A fast to help others could also mean that you fast on behalf of the needs that others are facing. Nehemiah learned that the Jewish remnant in Jerusalem that survived the exile was in great need. He says,

> *"When I heard these things, I sat down and wept. For some days I mourned and fasted and prayed before the God of heaven."* (Nehemiah 1:4)

Through his prayer and fasting, God opened the way for Nehemiah to go to his people and meet their needs. Fast with acts of mercy or fast for the relief of someone in need. Either way it is a good fast done for the needs of others.

Fasting for transformation

It's good when you fast to change your own life. Isaiah 58:9 speaks of a people who fast in order to do away with the pointing finger or malicious talk. Through their fast they recognize their bad behavior, repent and seek God to change their lives. Fast to discover the secret and hidden sins of you life. Fasting can be the means by which you see the true condition of your soul. Rees Howells tells how even his angry resistance to enter a fast brought him to a place of seeing his selfish appetites. "I didn't know such a lust was in me," he said, "my agitation was the proof of the grip it had on me. If the thing had no power over me, why did I argue about it?"[4] After you discover the sins in your life, fast to repent. Even Ahab, one of the most evil persons in the Bible, finds a gracious divine response when he repents of his sin through fasting (1 Kings 21:27).

Fast for change in your behavior. Possibly this was what Paul was doing when he went into a three day waterless fast after his conversion (Acts 9:9). Fasting is a means by which the grace of God can be released into your life in greater doses to bring significant change to your behavior. So fast for change!

The key is essential

Here is the bad news. No amount of our human ingenuity can pry open the doors to the needed resources of the kingdom. If it is up to our abilities, these doors will stay locked up forever. But there is also good news. A key exists that opens these doors. The key is fasting. But it is not any kind of fasting. Only a good fast is the master key that releases these much-needed resources of the kingdom of God.

Fast to obey God, defeat the enemy, help others and change yourself. If you fast the good fast, then God will trust you with the master key. The master key opens every door in God's storehouse.

Notes

1. John Wesley, *Wesley's 52 Standard Sermons* (Salem: Schmul Pub. 1988) p. 285
2. G.E.H. Palmer, Philip Sherrard and Kallistos Ware – translators, *The Philokalia* (Boston: Faber and Faber, 1979), Vol. 1, p. 164
3. Randy Clarke, compiler, *Power Holiness and Evangelism* (Shippensburg: Destiny Image, 1999) p. 109
4. Norman Grubb, *Rees Howells Intercessor* (Fort Washington: Christian Literature Crusade, 1952) p. 56

Chapter 4

The Door to Revelation

"Then your light will break forth like the dawn."
(Isaiah 58:8)

Knowledge that Surpasses Knowledge

When Paul became a believer he saw a brilliant blast of revelation on the Damascus road. Then he descended into total darkness. He went blind. People had to lead him as he stumbled around. That's an accurate picture of a lot of believers. They have a wonderful blast of revelation that Jesus is their Savior and then they enter a dark world of little revelation. Without revelation they stumble around in their spiritual lives.

In Paul's letter to the Ephesians he records two prayers for the church. In these prayers he specifically asks God three times to give the believers revelation (Ephesians 1:17–18; 3:19). He prays for the Spirit of revelation and wisdom. He also asks that the eyes of the people's hearts will be enlightened. Finally, Paul prays that the church might know the love of Jesus that surpasses knowledge. This final petition is a good definition of revelation. Revelation is knowledge from God that surpasses human knowledge. It is a trans-rational experience where God brings knowledge to your spirit. It isn't irrational but trans-rational. It transcends the rational thought processes. Revelation is absolutely essential. Without it you will be spiritually blind and stumble around in your faith. This is the reason Paul prays for the eyes of the heart to be opened.

How do you get revelation? Seek God's voice through faith, intimacy with Jesus and openness to the Holy Spirit. Believe for and expect revelation. In addition to these acts of faith, fasting opens the door to revelation. Isaiah 58:8 says that after you fast, *"your light will break forth like the dawn."* That's what happened to Paul. When he was blind, he fasted for three days and the Lord gave him a vision of Ananias coming to restore his sight (Acts 9:12). A vision enlightened the eyes of Paul's heart so he would receive Ananias to open his physical eyes. There are three levels of revelation you should seek. Fasting helps God's light of revelation to rise like the dawn.

Illumination through the Word

Revelation is God's illumination. Illumination is when God's Word comes to your spirit. The primary place you get divine illumination is through reading the Bible because it is inspired. Although the Bible is inspired, reading the Bible doesn't mean you automatically get a word from the Lord. You could simply get information about doctrine, prophecies, history or laws. There is nothing wrong with that. It is important information. But you need more.

I went to a liberal seminary where some professors who pored over the Scriptures did not get revelation. They only got information to support their theories of Biblical criticism. Reading the Bible didn't automatically bring them illumination. Just as God illuminated the authors of the books of Scripture when they wrote, so He must illuminate you when you read the Scriptures. The first illumination is called inspiration. The second is called revelation. God spoke into a person to record His Word and God also speaks into you as you read it.

So how should you read the Bible to get revelation? Read it in faith, expecting God to speak. And one way to turn up the light of revelation is through fasting. In my life the Bible never seems as alive as when I fast. One couple saw an immediate difference in their ability to receive revelation through the Bible when they started fasting one day a week. "God has opened our eyes to things that we have read before," they reported, "but have never seen specifically – it's as though ideas are just jumping out at us!"[1]

Fasting played an important role in giving us the inspired Word of God. Moses fasted for forty days before he received the illumination of the Ten Commandments (Exodus 34:28). Daniel fasted when he got inspired words of the end-times (Daniel 9:3). Paul, who wrote a significant part of the New Testament, said he fasted often (2 Corinthians 11:27). If fasting helped these men receive so much of the original inspiration of God's Word could it not release in you a present illumination from His Word?

Illumination through gifts

But the Bible is not the only place we get divine illumination. In 1 Corinthians 12:7–11 Paul lists the gifts of the Holy Spirit. He speaks of many of the revelatory gifts that come from divine illumination. The revelatory gifts are words of knowledge, words of wisdom, discernment of spirits, prophecy, tongues and interpretation of tongues. Paul is not speaking of the knowledge you get from your own rational processing of a situation. These spiritual gifts are direct revelations of the Holy Spirit into your human spirit. They are transrational words from God.

All revelatory words from the Holy Spirit must line up with God's written Word. That's why it is important that you read the Bible even as information. Always check your revelation against the Word of God.

Again, fasting turns up illumination through the gifts of the Holy Spirit. After Joel's three calls to fast he explains that the fruit of this fasting will be a wonderful outpouring of illumination on God's people.

> *"I will pour out my Spirit on all people,*
> *Your sons and daughters will prophesy,*
> *your old men will dream dreams,*
> *your young men will see visions."* (Joel 2:28)

Fasting helps bring illumination through the Bible and the gifts of the Holy Spirit.

Interpreting God's illumination

But sometimes an illumination from God is not enough. You can get a word from the Lord but you don't understand it. In that case the revelation you need is divine interpretation. Interpretation is getting a word from God about a word from God. Maybe you had an unusual dream or a vision. You know it is from God but you don't understand it. Possibly a verse or portion of the Bible jumps out at you. But you are not sure what God is saying through this word. There may be a word in tongues or a prophetic message that you don't fully understand. Ask the Lord for an interpretation. You don't want a word for word translation of what was spoken. Interpretation is different from translation. Seek an overall meaning of what God said.

Fasting increases interpretation

In the book of Daniel there were four Hebrews in Babylon who could interpret what God was saying through dreams and visions. Daniel 1:17 reports about Daniel, Hananiah, Mishael and Azariah saying,

> *"God gave knowledge and understanding of all kinds of literature and learning. And Daniel could understand visions and dreams of all kinds."*

Then verse 20 proclaims,

> *"In every matter of wisdom and understanding about which the king questioned them, he found them ten times better than all the magicians and enchanters in his whole kingdom."*

Remember that Babylon was an occult society. Magicians sought supernatural knowledge from their demon gods. But all their expertise in the occult could not compete with the light of God's interpretation that came through these four Hebrews.

The Queen of Babylon said,

> *"This man, Daniel . . . was found to have a keen mind and knowledge and understanding, and also the ability to interpret dreams, explain riddles and solve difficult problems."* (Daniel 5:12)

These interpretations came from God not from the intellectual abilities of the four Hebrew men. How did they turn up the light of God's interpretation? They fasted. In Daniel 1:12 we learn of a partial fast that all four men entered. Several other times you can read of Daniel fasting in order to receive revelation from the

Lord (Daniel 9:3 for instance). The light of divine interpretation is increased through fasting.

God's application

Revelation is illumination and interpretation but it is also application. You know God has spoken and you know what it means. But you don't know what to do with it. Wisdom is to know what to do with what God has given you. This wisdom comes from divine revelation.

Again, you get God's application through fasting. In Acts 13:2 the leaders of the church in Antioch were worshiping and fasting when God gave them a word. He told them to set Paul and Barnabas apart for the work to which He had called them. After the leaders received illumination for Paul and Barnabas to go, they fasted some more and laid hands on the two leaders. The Lord gave them an application, the first divine strategy for missions. How did they get it? It was through fasting.

During the great healing revival in the middle of the last century there was an anointed evangelist. God saved, healed and delivered many people through his ministry. But it wasn't always that way. In the beginning he had a call to heal the sick but did not know how. One day he asked his wife to lock him into the closet of their kitchen. He was determined to fast and pray until he heard from the Lord. After what seemed like days seeking God, the glory of the Lord suddenly filled the closet. It was so bright he thought his wife had opened the door. God began to give him clear steps he was to take to enter into his healing ministry. He found a pencil on the floor of the closet. He sharpened it with his teeth. Tearing off the flap to a cardboard box he began to write the eleven points of application that God gave him. This application led him into a ministry that eventually touched thousands with the gospel.[2]

The dark side of revelation

Unfortunately there is more to the story. This evangelist eventually fell into pride and isolation. When he died prematurely there was a lot of confusion about his faithfulness in the ministry. I share this sad part of the story to make a point. Revelation, no matter how great or powerful, does not guarantee infallibility. As a matter of fact, revelation can bring pride.

Paul says in 2 Corinthians 12:7,

> *"To keep me from becoming conceited because of these surpassingly great revelations, there was given me a thorn in my flesh, a messenger of Satan, to torment me."*

Protect yourself from the pride that can come with revelation. Revelation alone is not enough. It can be dangerous. Humility, honesty and relationship with others will protect you from being scorched with any pride. Then you can safely fast for the light of revelation to break forth like the dawn.

Notes

1. Basic Care Bulletin 4, *How To Discover the Rewards of Fasting* (Oak Brook: Medical Training Institute of America, 1990) p. 9
2. Robert Liardon, *God's Generals, Why They Succeeded and Why Some Failed* (Tulsa: Albury Publishing, 1996) pp. 407–410

Chapter 5

The Door to Healing

"And your healing will quickly appear."
"The LORD *... will strengthen your frame."*
(Isaiah 58:8, 11)

Natural or Supernatural

Several years ago Kerry, a good friend of mine, was suffering with hypoglycemia. That is an abnormally low level of glucose in the blood. It was a constant battle to keep his sugar-level under control. At times he would fast a little but it would get him so out of balance and sick that he had to break the fast. It took days to recover. I sensed that if Kerry would commit to a forty-day fast, the Lord would heal him. Generally I do not give that kind of advice to folks. After I told him, Kerry sought the Lord for two more confirmations. The Lord gave two more and an inner witness to do it.

When Kerry began he did not have the adverse effects he usually experienced. By the middle of the fast he was feeling better than he had felt for years. After the forty days of fasting, he was completely healed. Kerry said he never felt as good as he did then. He had forgotten what wholeness was like. Did the Lord heal Kerry by the natural strengthening of his body through fasting, or did the Lord heal him by the supernatural power that fasting and faith can bring? The answer is yes. Isaiah 58:8 says that fasting can bring supernatural healing. Verse 11 says that fasting can bring natural well-being. Fasting unlocks the door to both kinds of healing.

The fastest way to health

Physical health comes through fasting. The Lord has created your body to be strengthened through fasting. Paraclesus, a fifteenth-century physician, said,

> "Fasting is the greatest remedy, the physician within."[1]

Why is that the case?

Fasting and drinking a lot of liquids gives your body the needed opportunity to flush out all the poisons and toxins you have accumulated through years of eating and drinking. If you never changed the oil in your car but just kept adding to it when it was low, it would eventually clog up the engine. Oil gets dirty. It is not enough to keep putting new oil in the engine. The old oil must come out. Do you constantly put food and drink into your body but never cleanse it from the toxins that are accumulating?

Paul Braggs says,

> "Fasting gives the body a physiological rest and permits the body to become one hundred percent efficient in healing itself. Fasting under proper care is the fastest, and the safest way or means of regaining health ..."[2]

Fasting strengthens the immune system, relieves inflammation like arthritis, gets rid of toxins and breaks down plaque build up. In some cases it has been known to manage cancer, overcome obesity and enhance sensory perception. A lifestyle of fasting brings great physical benefits.[3] But fasting for health alone is not a biblical fast. In biblical fasting, good health is not the purpose. It is a benefit. The purpose of fasting is to engage the Lord in faith and experience His presence in fuller measure. If you set out solely to improve your health with fasting that's fine, but it is not a biblical fast. If you set out to engage the Lord in faith and your frame is strengthened as a result of your fast, then that is a biblical fast.

One couple discovered this surprising benefit on the eighth day of a fast. The wife wrote,

> "My husband woke up with no ringing in his right ear. He had had a ringing and partial deafness in the ear for 24 years due to a terrible accident in which he had been crushed under a four-ton forklift. His hearing is now restored, and the ringing is gone!"[4]

The intent of their fast was to engage the Lord in faith. Restored health was a benefit.

There is nothing wrong with growing healthy in your body as you grow healthy in your soul. Third John 2 says,

> *"I pray that you may enjoy good health and that all may go well with you, even as your soul is getting along well."*

Health is not the purpose of biblical fasting but it certainly is a great result.

Healing that comes quickly

Fasting in faith can also bring supernatural healing. Isaiah 58:8 describes a manifestation of healing that comes rapidly. It is a supernatural touch from God.

David speaks of this supernatural power to heal through fasting. In Psalm 35:13 he says,

> *"Yet when they were ill, I put on sackcloth and humbled myself with fasting."*

Here David prayed and fasted for the healing of other people who were ill. Since he was fasting for others he saw it as a means for supernatural healing. David also fasted for healing in 2 Samuel 12:15–18. It was for his son who was born out of his adulterous relationship with Bathsheba. The child became ill through the judgment of God against David. David fasted and prayed for healing. But the son died. Although there was no healing, this verse gives us insight into how David fasted and prayed for the sick.

David was earnest in his fast. He saw fasting coupled with prayer as important when believing for healing even though the fasting cost him. He was also focused. He gave himself to the prayer and fasting totally. He spent nights on the floor. Even when others were pleading with him to stop, relax and eat, he continued in his fast.

He was specific in his fast. David fasted for the healing of his son. After his son died, he stopped the fast and returned to life as normal. The servant asked him why he quit fasting after his son died. David informed the servant he wasn't fasting to grieve over his son's death or to keep repenting of his sin. His one purpose in fasting was for his son's healing. David's fast was earnest, focused and specific.

A conqueror in Jesus' name

Guy Bevington, an evangelist in the early part of the twentieth century, fasted like David. Once he was in

Cleveland, Ohio and received a letter from the wife of an old friend in Chattanooga. In the letter she told how her husband was dying. She wrote, "By the time you get this letter, Mr. Allen will be buried."

Bevington took the letter into his prayer room and asked that no one bother him. He began to fast and pray. He prayed for eleven hours just to see if his friend was still alive. Bevington explained that because he had so much on his mind it took him that long just to get the voice of God. The Lord gave him a vision in which he saw Mr. Allen lying like a dead man completely white. But Bevington was not allowed to break the vision so he lay on the floor for five more minutes until he saw Mr. Allen raise his right hand and smile. Knowing he was still alive through this vision, Guy Bevington said, "Amen, Lord, now for his healing." He prayed for another nine hours to get God's will for healing Mr. Allen. That was twenty hours on his face before God. It took him just forty-six more hours to see his friend a healed man. Bevington said, "After laying in the dark room for 66 hours, I could walk out a conqueror in the name of Jesus."

Mr. Allen was healed and immediately asked his wife if she had written to Bevington. When she told him she had, he said, "Well he has prayed through for me and I am healed." Guy Bevington was earnest, focused and specific in his fasting for healing.[5]

Facets of divine healing

When you fast for healing, it can take place in many areas of your life. One area is in your body or in the body of someone you love. Fast and pray for your loved one or for yourself. God can touch the human body and make it whole.

Fasting can be for the healing of your soul. God restores the soul though inner healing and deliverance.

In Mark 9:29 Jesus speaks of the importance of wholehearted prayer, which can include fasting, to bring deliverance to people. Fasting brings inner healing.

The human spirit also needs healing. Those people not born again are dead in their human spirit. Pray for their salvation with fasting. They need the spiritual healing that will bring their dead spirits to life.

Finally fast for the healing of communities. Churches, cities or even nations need corporate healing. The people of Nineveh entered into a fast and their city was healed from corporate sin (Jonah 3:6–10).

Fasting for healing of people and the land

In 1947 Franklin Hall wrote a book entitled *Atomic Power With God Through Fasting and Prayer.* It became a catalyst for many people to do a forty-day fast for healing and revival. Over the next five years the great healing revivals erupted throughout the United States. Many of these healing evangelists saw powerful miracles as they followed the fasting directions that Hall laid out in his book. Revivals also came for the healing of souls and the healing of the land. The "Latter Rain" revival invaded the United States out of Canada in 1948. Billy Graham's ministry began a year later. In 1950 Asbury College experienced a powerful move of God. After the call to fast went out from Franklin Hall's book "47 to 50 massive revival tremors shook the earth."[6]

The quick turn around that can only come by the supernatural power of God is found behind the door of healing. One key that unlocks this door is fasting.

Notes

1. Paul Bragg, *The Miracle of Fasting* (Santa Barbara: Health Science, 1996) cover

2. Ibid, p. 145
3. Basic Care Bulletin 4, *How To Discover the Rewards of Fasting* (Oak Brook: Medical Training Institute of America, 1990) pp. 7–12
4. Ibid, p. 9
5. G.C. Bevington, *Remarkable Incidents and Modern Miracles through Prayer and Faith* (Kokomo: New Book Room) pp. 72, 78
6. Lou Engle, *Atomic Power Through Fasting and Prayer*, Spread the Fire, December 1996, p. 13

Chapter 6

The Door to Holiness

"Then your righteousness will go before you."
(Isaiah 58:8)

Spiritual Grace Injector

Isaiah says that if you fast, *"then your righteousness will go before you"* (Isaiah 58:8). Righteousness will work itself out in your life so that people see holiness. But fasting doesn't make you holy. Only the Holy Spirit can do that. When you are filled with the Holy Spirit the fire of God transforms your human will so that you can consistently and passionately choose for God. The Holy Spirit begins to manifest within you the character of Jesus.

If only the Holy Spirit makes you holy, how is fasting a key to holiness? When you couple fasting with another spiritual dynamic, whether it is prayer, worship or brokenness, that spiritual dynamic moves into a deeper dimension. Couple fasting with the baptism in the Holy Spirit and it intensifies the work of the Spirit in your life. Fasting becomes the fuel injector for the fire of the Holy Spirit! It brings high performance to the work of sanctification.

Ceasing to eat won't make you holy. But fasting will enhance your transformation by the Holy Spirit when you combine it with faith. Believe the Holy Spirit to infuse a greater measure of His power into your life. Fasting will then become a spiritual grace injector. Without faith and Spirit baptism, however, fasting for holiness is a sterile discipline. Try to become holy with a faithless fast and you will end up on a treadmill of legalism. You won't become holy. You'll become worn out.

Fast in faith. Believe the Holy Spirit to meet you. His grace will be injected in greater intensity. The Holy Spirit will increasingly transform three selfish areas.

Choose for God

Fasting and faith work with the Holy Spirit to overcome self-indulgence. That is important because self-indulgence keeps you from choosing God's will. A brief sampling of biblical history shows the danger of indulgence with food. Sin came into the world when Adam and Eve chose pleasures through eating a forbidden fruit instead of obeying God. Esau lost a godly inheritance when he gave into self-indulgence and traded his inheritance for a meal. The Hebrews refused to follow God because they were in bondage to the foods of Egypt (Genesis 3:6; 25:29–34; Exodus 16:3). It is easier to choose for selfish pleasures than to choose God's will. If you don't show restraint toward self-indulgence you destroy kingdom destinies, lose godly inheritances and miss promises.

Here is the good news. The constant pull toward self-indulgence can be overcome! Through baptism in the Holy Spirit the power of God can so transform your will that you choose for God's pleasure instead of self-indulgence. When you regularly add fasting to fullness, it intensifies the measure of grace that moves you to choose for God. It doesn't make you choose for God. It empowers you so you are able to passionately choose His will.

Jesus knew the power of this divine recipe. He was filled with the Holy Spirit in the Jordan. He then entered a forty-day fast in the desert. When the enemy tried to get him to come into self-indulgence and miss God's greater purpose, Jesus was able to resist. He chose for God. Jesus thundered back at the Devil who tried to tempt him with food saying,

> *"Man does not live on bread alone, but on every word that comes from the mouth of God."* (Matthew 4:4)

One couple discovered the power of fasting for holiness. They wrote,

> "Since we started fasting once a week, we have both noticed that we have more victory over temptations which we normally may have given in to."[1]

God wants you to enjoy some of the pleasures of this world but not at the expense of missing His will. Only the Holy Spirit can empower you to choose against your self-indulgence and for the will of God. Fasting brings the sanctifying fire of the Holy Spirit to a white heat.

Thinking right

Not only is self-indulgence a problem but also self-deception. If self-indulgence keeps you from choosing right, self-deception keeps you from thinking right. There is a deceptive grid over the human mind that comes through the curse of sin. It causes you to see yourself as the center of life. It convinces you that you are strong. You are able to run your life. You can keep things together. And God is somewhere on the periphery of your life. Self-deception creates the illusion of self-importance.

The Holy Spirit not only wants you to choose differently, He wants you to think differently. Paul says in Romans 12:2,

> *"Do not conform any longer to the pattern of this world, but be transformed by the renewing of your mind. Then you will be able to test and approve what God's will is – his good, pleasing and perfect will."*

When the Holy Spirit fills you He begins to renew your mind with new thoughts. He gives you a new perspective that is God-centered in place of self-centered. Fasting plays a role in helping the Holy Spirit to transform your mind.

I'll be honest. I don't like to fast. I don't feel good when I fast. I get headaches. Many times I feel weak, jumpy and depressed. But that is God's way of showing me who I really am. He takes off the self-deception and shows me I am not the center of the world. In myself, I am weak. I have been made something only by the grace of God. God is the center of life, not me. When I empty myself of food, I not only know I am weak, I experience it. There are some spiritual truths you must experience. Not all these spiritual experiences are enjoyable. You need to experience how weak and fragile you are so that you know how strong and faithful God is. Fasting brings you to weakness and God always meets you in that weakness. It dismantles the grid of deception and brings you to a greater dependency on the Lord. John Wesley saw the power in transforming the minds of his people through fasting. "The reason why the Methodists in general do not live in this salvation is," he said, "there is too little fasting and self-denial and too little self-examination."[2]

Taking deception off the church

William Duma was praying for his congregation when he sensed self-deception was in his church. He called all his leaders to fast and pray before the next communion to see if there was any deception in their lives. During the service Duma felt the power of the Holy Spirit flowing through the church. When he served the communion one of the leaders who had refused to fast and pray, dropped the plate of bread and fell to the ground. He was assisted to another room.

The church was afraid. There was a sense that God's holy presence was brooding over the service. Later the shaken leader confessed to Pastor Duma his hypocrisy and deception. He told of misconduct in his work and his private life. He sought the forgiveness of Jesus and his fellow believers. Duma said, "The spiritual life and power of the church deepened most perceptibly. It seemed ever clearer to me that what Christians need – and need acutely – is a deep hunger for God."[3]

The Holy Spirit renews your mind and the mind of your church. The Holy Spirit uses fasting to transform the way you think. He gives you the mind of Christ instead of a self-deceived mind.

Legalism or addiction

The Holy Spirit also empowers you to overcome self-gratification. Your body craves gratification, whether it is with food, sex, sleep or comfort. If these cravings are not restrained and tamed, the appetites of your body will control your life. Unrestrained self-gratification opens the door through your body to bondage by the enemy.

That is why Paul speaks over and over again of taming those passions. In Romans 13:14 Paul says, *"do not think about how to gratify the flesh"* (KJV). He tells the believers in Colossians 3:5 to *"mortify your members."* In other words, keep your body under control. In 1 Corinthians 9:27 Paul compares himself to an athlete who keeps his body disciplined. He must make it a servant to his spirit.[4]

Be proactive in keeping your body under control or Satan will use your body to control you with addictions and habits. Some believers try to control their bodies through the chains of legalism. They so tie down their body with rules, regulations and disciplines that they don't have any gratification. They believe that refusing all gratification will protect them from a bondage to self-gratification. But God created the hungers of your body. It is not that they are bad in themselves. But without restraint they will bind you with the ropes and chains of addiction.

Are these the only two options? Either bind yourself with legalism or bind yourself with addictions? There is another way. The Holy Spirit can empower you with His fullness. He can make you so passionate for Jesus Christ that all your other passions take second place. By fasting you can work with the Holy Spirit for a greater infusion of this passion for Jesus. Fasting arrests the appetite for food, sex and sleep. Because food feeds all the desires of your body, fasting curbs them. Fasting is the enemy of self-gratification. It gives the Holy Spirit space to minister into you more of His holy fire.

Penetration by fire

St. Simeon speaks of this sanctifying work. He explains,

> "Can he, who has in his heart the Divine fire of the Holy Spirit burning naked, not be set on fire, not

> shine and glitter and not take on the radiance of the Deity in the degree of his purification and penetration by fire? For penetration by fire follows upon purification of the heart, and again purification of heart follows upon penetration by fire."[5]

One of the great helps in this penetration by fire is a fasting lifestyle. This is a part of the sanctifying process. Through this daily walking in the Spirit you begin to choose like Jesus, think like Jesus and feel like Jesus. Fasting is the grace injector for the sanctifying fire of the Holy Spirit. As you fast in faith, the Holy Spirit accomplishes great transformations in your will, mind and body. He causes your righteousness to go before you.

Notes

1. Basic Care Bulletin 4, *How To Discover the Rewards of Fasting* (Oak Brook: Medical Training Institute of America, 1990) p. 9
2. Arthur Wallis, *God's Chosen Fast* (Pennsylvania: Christian Literature Crusade, 1968) p. 87
3. Mary Garnett, *Take Your Glory Lord* (Kent: Sovereign World, 2000) pp. 32, 33
4. David Smith, *Fasting A Neglected Discipline* (Chichester: New Wine Press, 1954) p. 44
5. E. Kadloubovsky and G.E.H. Palmer – translators, *Writings from the Philokalia on Prayer of the Heart* (Boston: Faber and Faber, 1951) pp. 118–119

Chapter 7

The Door to Protection

"Then . . . the glory of the LORD will be your rear guard."
(Isaiah 58:8)

A Dangerous Journey

Ezra and 1,754 men, women and children who had been exiled in Babylon stood on the country's border getting ready to journey back to their home, Jerusalem, to resettle there. The trip would be a long journey of five months. They were to travel through an ungoverned region filled with dangerous tribes and hostile bandits. To make matters worse they were carrying with them treasures to help in the resettlement and rebuilding of Jerusalem that were worth between three and four million dollars!

This is a picture of people who need protection. And it really is a similar picture of all believers. You too are on a long journey to your heavenly home through this world. The Bible says you are traveling through this present evil age. It is filled with a supernatural enemy of God and demonic bandits, who are determined to kill, steal and destroy. And you carry with you the very treasures of the kingdom of God. That is why Jesus encouraged His disciples to pray, *"Deliver us from evil one"* (Matthew 6:13). It is also why Jesus prayed for His disciples in John 17:15, *"Protect them from the evil one."* Where do you get protection for your journey? Look back at Ezra. Instead of relying on an escort from Babylon to protect him, he relied on someone more reliable: Almighty God. Ezra called the people to fast and pray for divine protection. He testified at the end of the journey,

> *"The hand of our God was on us, and he protected us from enemies and bandits along the way."* (Ezra 8:31)

Glory and protection

Fasting unlocks the door to divine protection over your life. Isaiah 58:8 says that when you enter a good fast *"then the glory of the LORD will be your rear guard."* The Isaiah passage refers to a time in Israel's history when the armies of Egypt were closing in to slaughter over a million Hebrews cornered by the Red Sea. Then the glory of the Lord guiding the Israelites as a pillar of cloud moved from the front of the great crowd to the rear. It became a guard between the Hebrews and the fury of the Egyptian army (Exodus 14:5–20).

Exodus 14:20 reads,

> *"Throughout the night the cloud brought darkness to the one side and light to the other; so neither went near the other all night long."*

In other words, the glory of the Lord became their rear guard. The Bible contains many accounts of fasting that brings divine protection. If you are sensing you are under attack or in a vulnerable place spiritually, look at the two ways the glory of God brings protection. Then examine how fasting releases the glory of God.

Scrambling the enemy's schemes

One way God's glory protects is to keep evil from you. He brings darkness to the side of evil so it can't get at you. Just as the glory of the Lord brought confusion to the army of Egypt, He will scramble the schemes of the enemy that are planned against you.

King Jehoshaphat, the King of Judah, needed that kind of help. He had just learned that several enemy nations had joined themselves together to form a super-army. Their purpose was to destroy Judah. The people of Judah didn't have what was needed to defeat this massive assault. So the King called the men, women and children to join him in Jerusalem for a fast. When they assembled together he prayed to God, *"We do not know what to do, but our eyes are upon you"* (2 Chronicles 20:12).

Because of Judah's fasting and prayer three things were set in motion. First, the Holy Spirit moved on Jahaziel to prophesy, *"Do not be afraid or discouraged because of this vast army. For the battle is not yours, but God's"* (2 Chronicles 20:15). Second, because the people heard from the Lord in this prophetic promise they exploded in worship to God until they spilled out of the city toward the approaching armies. Third, as they praised God, His glory brought confusion to the invading armies so that the enemy troops turned on each other and totally annihilated themselves (2 Chronicles 20:1–30).

It is obvious that this warfare against Judah was not just natural but also supernatural. The people of Israel were not only being attacked outwardly by a massive army, but inwardly by fear. Through their fasting, God dispelled the fear with a prophetic word and with praise. Then He destroyed the outward threat supernaturally by bringing the enemy troops into confusion. If Judah had given into their fears they would have been destroyed. Instead, a national crisis turned into revival!

Olga Robertson ministered for years in the Muntinlupa Prison in the Philippines. She would go into cells with two hundred inmates. Here were prisoners who had committed murder and rape. They were severely demonized. Olga went in with great courage. She had no fear and the men knew it. What was her secret? "I could never do this work," she said, "if I didn't fast one day a week. Many of these men have demons and I need the power of God when I minister."[1] Fasting brings inward protection and outward protection with supernatural power.

Are you facing an ongoing attack of the enemy or great crises on the horizon of your life? Fast and pray and watch the glory of the Lord deliver you from both the inward and outward attacks of evil.

Know where to step

God not only keeps evil from you, He keeps you from evil. In the story of the pillar of cloud becoming Israel's rear guard, while darkness came to the Egyptian army light came to the children of Israel. God brought light to the Hebrew people so they could see the presence of the enemy troops and not wander off into their camp. This present evil age is a minefield of satanic deception to bring you to spiritual defeat. But divine protection brings light to your spirit so you know how to miss all the dangers, snares and traps. You must know where to step.

Esther found herself in a similar minefield. She desperately needed God's light. Esther was a humble Hebrew women exiled in Persia. The King of Persia, not knowing she was a Hebrew, chose her to be his wife, the Queen. At this time there was a plot by an evil man in the government to exterminate the entire Jewish race. Because of Esther's access to the King she was the only one who could stop this holocaust. But there was a problem. Royal protocol forbade Esther to approach the King with a request – for this she would more than likely be put to death!

Esther spread the word through her cousin, Mordecai, to have all the Jews enter an extreme fast: no water and no food, for three days. Due to the fast three things happened. First, when Esther approached the King he welcomed her with great love. Second, God gave Esther a unique strategy to help the King see this evil plot against the Jews. Finally, God moved upon the heart of the King and the evil man to unconsciously play into Esther's strategy for deliverance. Ultimately the King executed the man who hatched the plan to kill the Jews (Esther 1–8).

The glory of the Lord gives you light so you receive divine strategies that overcome demonic schemes and bring you to victory. The glory of God also infuses you with holiness so the enemy has no foothold to bring you down with temptation. Fasting releases greater measures of God's glory to keep you from evil.

The Lord will help you

At a camp meeting in Brown City, Michigan I had been teaching on fasting. After the session, Sarah Hazard, the humble wife of a farmer, told me she had done three fasts of forty days. During one of those fasts, while in her kitchen, the Lord clearly said, "I, the Lord, will help thee." Not long after this word she heard an explosion outside the house. Again, the Lord said, "I will help thee." Sarah looked out to see fire billowing up from their tractor near the barn. Her husband was running from the fire with no clothes on. His clothes had caught fire and he had pulled them off. She ran out with something for him to put on.

As they were running from the fire Sarah's husband asked her, "What are we going to do if we lose our tractor?" She turned to him and said, "The Lord will help us." No sooner had she said it than he began to shout, "Look! Look!" Sarah turned to see the fire go back into the oil drum and gas can sitting near the tractor. It receded into the container and went out. When Sarah later checked the gas can it was still half full. Her husband was badly burned on the back of his legs. Even though the doctor told him he would need skin grafts his legs healed completely and all he had was a little scar on his arm. The tractor was up and running after buying a five dollar part that had been melted.

Does this mean that if you fast and pray you will always be protected from harm? No. Paul fasted and prayed often and still took hits from the enemy at times. He was after all constantly on the front lines. But he may have taken even more hits if he hadn't fasted for protection. This is a present evil age and you do have an enemy out there. You also have a powerful God who moves on your behalf to protect you as you call out to Him. Fast to increase the glory of the Lord. The enemy will be confused and you will be enlightened.

Note

1. Gwen Shaw, *Your Appointment With God* (Jasper: End-Time Handmaidens, Inc., 1977) p. 38

Chapter 8

The Door to Answers

"Then you will call, and the LORD will answer."
(Isaiah 58:9)

When There Is No Answer

What do you do when you pray and no answer comes? Shift into whole-hearted prayer. This is extreme praying. In Jeremiah 29:13 God says,

> *"You will seek me and find me when you seek me with all your heart."*

What happens in whole-hearted praying? In Joel 2:12 God explains, *"Return to me with all your heart."* Then He defines what that includes when He says, *"with fasting, weeping and mourning."* When you call on the Lord out of the depth of your being with fasting then *"the LORD will answer"* (Isaiah 58:9). Have you ever prayed with your whole heart? That is when eating, sleeping, social contacts and emotional comfort are put on hold until the answer comes. This type of prayer is essential to get answers in some difficult circumstances that block God's response.

Change self-dependence

Self-dependency keeps you from faith. Without faith God's answers will not come. Prayer with your whole heart transforms your attitude. It changes you from self-dependence to dependence on God. Fast and believe to depend on God. Self-dependence can be deceptive. It doesn't have to be an obnoxious fixation on your ego. You might trust in your hate of sin, zeal for holiness or passion for ministry. Still you trust in your abilities instead of in God.

Before Israel had a king the tribe of Benjamin committed a horrible act of brutality and rebelled against the rest of the nation. The other tribes of Israel gathered nearly a half million troops to put down the Benjamites' rebellion. The Lord instructed Israel to send the strong troops of Judah in first. But the Benjamites slaughtered twenty-two thousand of Judah's troops in the first military engagement. Next the Lord instructed the other tribes to send in their troops. In the second battle Israel lost eighteen thousand men. After these heavy losses the Israelites went before the Lord for a whole day of fasting and weeping. God promised victory. When the Israelites attacked again, they routed the Benjamites, killing twenty-five thousand of their troops. The rebellion was over (Judges 20:1–48).

What was the difference between the first two attacks and the last attack? Fasting changed Israel's attitude. Before the fast the people depended on their anger against the Benjamites and their zeal for the nation. After the fast and the two defeats they depended on the Lord for victory.

Hudson Taylor found a group of Chinese Christians that fasted often. He said,

> "They recognize that this fasting, which so many dislike, which requires faith in God, since it makes

> one feel weak and poorly, is really a divinely appointed means of grace. Perhaps the greatest hindrance to our work is our own imagined strength; and in fasting we learn what poor, weak creatures we are."[1]

Fasting changes your imagined strength to a dependence on God's strength. When your attitude changes and you get in faith, the answer of God comes.

Break Satan's resistance

Answers also don't come because of demonic blockades that keep out God's supplies. Fast to change the enemy. When you pray with your whole heart these demonic powers shift from resistance into retreat.

Daniel was exiled in a land swarming with demonic activity. One day he made a request of God. The Lord heard Daniel and immediately responded with an answer. But a strong demonic power over the region, called the Prince of the Kingdom of Persia, resisted the heavenly messenger sent to Daniel with the answer. Meanwhile, Daniel entered a twenty-one-day fast during this demonic interference. Because Daniel prayed with his whole heart, God sent an angelic reinforcement to overcome the resistance. The answer to Daniel's prayer came twenty-one days later than expected, but it finally arrived. If Daniel had not entered into his fast the ruling principality over Persia could have blocked the answer Daniel was seeking (Daniel 10:1–21).

Demonic powers war against the answers God has for you. They always run interference. They resist evangelism, missions and regional transformation. The heavenly messenger informed Daniel that when he was through overcoming the Prince of Persia, the Prince of Greece would come next (Daniel 10:20). Satanic powers are lining up to interfere with God's work in the world. But you are part of God's resistance movement behind enemy lines. Whole-hearted praying breaks demonic interference so that God's supplies get through.

Almolonga, Guatemala, was a town behind a massive demonic blockade. Alcoholism, immorality and abuse were common. Evangelists were chased away. Churches were weak and few. A local deity empowered demonic interference over the region. One church began to pray behind enemy lines with their whole heart. People that worshiped the local deity got saved and delivered. Other people were healed. Years of whole-hearted prayers overcame the satanic blockade. There are now nearly twenty-five evangelical churches. Four of them have a thousand members or more. Recently twelve thousand to fifteen thousand of a population of eighteen thousand gathered in the market square to pray. The jail is empty, bars are disappearing and people are prospering under God's blessings. A secular periodical, *Cronica Seminal*, reports,

> "The evangelical church ... constitutes the most significant force for religious change in the highlands of Guatemala since the Spanish conquest."[2]

Fast for divine conquest over demonic resistance. You can help bring the answers of God through enemy lines.

God wants a friend

Answers will not come when God's righteous anger is against a sinful and stubborn people. God doesn't send His blessings on people under His judgment. The only hope for getting God's answers is whole-hearted prayer. Prayer and fasting change God's heart. But don't get too proud, thinking you have the power to change God.

This only happens because God designed a loophole of mercy. Think of it. God welcomes you into His sovereignty to change His heart from anger to mercy.

When people sin, God has established three ways to respond. First, He can punish or destroy them with His righteous anger. Second, if people repent He can forgive them. He also has a third response. If people remain stubborn and don't repent God can still show mercy. But there must be an intercessor who uses this loophole of mercy through whole-hearted praying.[3] God looks for a friend to change His heart from anger to mercy. Isaiah 59:16 says that when God *"saw that there was no-one, he was appalled that there was no-one to intervene."* God is speechless when He looks and can't find anyone to use this loophole of mercy on behalf of people under His judgment.

God was furious when the Hebrews worshiped the golden calf. He informed Moses that He was going to destroy all the Hebrews. He was done with their rebellion. Moses began praying with all His heart, fasting forty days and forty nights. During this time Moses preached at God about the honor of His name, reminded God of His promises and pleaded with Him for a glimpse of His glory. God repented of destroying the Hebrews but told Moses He would not go with Moses and the Hebrews into the Promised Land. Moses boldly responded to God declaring, "I am not going in without you" (Exodus 33:15). God then changed and said He was willing to go in with His friend Moses but not with the Hebrews. Moses then informed God that he wasn't going in without the Hebrews. God finally agreed to go in with both Moses and the people. Moses pressed God harder for a divine covenant. Moses wanted a commitment from God that He would be the God of the Hebrews. He got it (Exodus 32–34; Deuteronomy 9:7–29).

In the forty days that Moses wrestled with God, God's

heart changed from anger to mercy. The Lord had a friend who was bold and reverent before Him. God said to Moses,

> *"I will do the very thing you have asked, because I am pleased with you and I know you by name."*
> (Exodus 33:17)

God loves an intercessor who engages Him as a friend to change His heart.

God's heart changed in an afternoon

The American evangelist, D.L. Moody, visited London and was unexpectedly invited to preach a morning service in a local church. It was a dead and cold church. Absolutely nothing happened in the service. That evening Moody preached again at the same church. God's Spirit was powerfully present. Many of the people responded to his invitation to receive Christ. Moody eventually spent ten days at the church and saw over four hundred people come to the Lord.

Why was there such a change from the morning service to the evening service? For some months a woman in the church who was confined to bed because of sickness had prayed for revival to come. Long before Moody came to London, she read of his ministry in America. She secretly prayed that God would send this evangelist to her church. When her sister returned from the morning service and informed her that an unknown and unexpected guest named D.L. Moody had preached, the intercessor turned pale and said, "God has heard my prayer." She spent the afternoon fasting and praying. She changed the Lord's anger against a cold rebellious church to mercy. Revival fire fell that night. Moody believed that one meeting opened the door for him to later return to England where thousands of people were saved and revival exploded across the nation.[4]

You too can open the door to God's answers when you pray and fast to change His heart. When it changes there is no stopping the flood of His mercies. Whether whole-hearted prayers change your attitude, the dynamics of spiritual warfare or the heart of God, things begin to happen. Call on the Lord with all your heart and His answers will come.

Notes

1. Maynard G. James, *The Practice of Fasting,* Dayspring, Nov.–Dec. 1964, p. 31
2. George Otis, Jr, *Informed Intercessors* (Ventura: Renew Books, 1999) pp. 18–23
3. Zacharias Tanee Fomum, *The Art of Intercession* (Mumbai: Crossroads Communication, 1996) pp. 23–24
4. A.P. Fitt, *The Shorter Life of D.L. Moody* (Chicago: Moody Press) pp. 68–70

Chapter 9

The Door to Presence

"You will cry for help and he will say: Here am I."
(Isaiah 58:9)

Jesus on Fasting

One of the most significant teachings Jesus gave about fasting is in Mark 2:18–22. The disciples of the Pharisees and John the Baptist were fasting but Jesus' disciples were not. Some people wanted to know why Jesus' disciples were not fasting like these other groups. In response Jesus reveals three truths.

First, His disciples didn't need to fast then. Since fasting to most Jews in this time was for grief over sin or loss, Jesus made the point that for His disciples it was not a time of sadness but of celebration. The bridegroom was with them. The kingdom of God was breaking into the world. It was a time for feasting not fasting. This was a wedding party not a funeral wake.

Second, there would be a day when His disciples would fast. When would this time be? When the bridegroom was taken from them. When Jesus was no longer physically present among His disciples, then they would fast.

Third, when this day came it would bring with it a new purpose in fasting. Previously the main purpose for fasting was for repentance and grief. But for Jesus' disciples, when He was no longer physically with them, fasting would primarily be for spiritual fellowship with Jesus.

Fasting enhances communion

Here, Jesus speaks of a new-wineskin fasting. He makes the point that new ways of doing things (new wineskins) are important for new works of God (fresh wine). The newest and greatest purpose for fasting in the kingdom of God is for communion with your absent bridegroom, the exalted Christ. First Peter 1:8–9 says,

> *"Though you have not seen him, you love him; and even though you do not see him now, you believe in him and are filled with an inexpressible and glorious joy, for you are receiving the goal of your faith, the salvation of your souls."*

The physical, visible presence of your bridegroom is no longer with you. In these days He can only be known according to the Spirit.

Fasting is not the reason you have spiritual fellowship with Jesus. Redemption is. Because your sins are forgiven and you have been born of the Spirit, you now can experience Jesus spiritually. Although fasting isn't the reason for spiritual communion, it does enhance your experience of the Lord. Isaiah 58:9 says that through your fasting you can have a clear sense of the Lord's presence. *"Here am I"* is His word to you.

After an extended fast one woman in Cameroon had an experience where she heard the audible voice of her absent bridegroom. She said,

> "The Eternal One told me in my ears, 'I love you.' I knew that the Eternal One loved me. But hearing Him tell me this directly was simply marvelous. My life has never been the same. The 'I love you' of the Lord Jesus was very beautiful. It has changed everything."[1]

You too can commune with your absent bridegroom. Fasting can be a means of strengthening your experience of the Lord in two ways.

Communion through worship

First, come to the Lord through worship. Worship is focusing your affections on the exalted Lord Jesus Christ. As you worship Jesus, you come into His presence. This communion with the Lord doesn't automatically happen because you sing words written in a hymnal or shown on a screen. Maybe you have worshiped but you didn't engage the Lord. You have to be intentional in going after Jesus. In 2 Corinthians 4:18 Paul says,

> *"So we fix our eyes not on what is seen, but on what is unseen."*

The way to the unseen presence of your absent Lord is to fix your heart on Him. Like a Cruise missile, fix onto the target of your affections dodging all the barriers and dips and curves that stand between you and Him. This focus of passion brings you into His spiritual presence.

Biblically, it is evident that fasting is an important way to come to Jesus in worship. Luke 2:37 says that Anna, *"never left the temple but worshiped day and night, fasting and praying."* In Acts 13:2 the Holy Spirit speaks to the leaders in the church *"while they were worshiping the Lord and fasting."* Also Nehemiah 9:1–3 reports that the Israelites worshiped the Lord while fasting.

Some early church fathers also spoke of worshiping the Lord through fasting. St. Diadochos, who lived four hundred years after Christ's ascension, explained,

> "We shall surely come to experience immaterial perception if by our labors we refine our material nature."[2]

Fasting is one way you refine your material nature.

Why does fasting sharpen your focus on the Lord Jesus Christ? Quite simply, food dulls your spiritual perception. Deuteronomy 6:11–12 says,

> *"...when you eat and are satisfied be careful that you do not forget the LORD."*

And Deuteronomy 8:10, 14 says,

> *"When you have eaten and are satisfied ... then your heart will become proud and you will forget the LORD your God."*

Overload your stomach and you dull your spirit so it loses the capacity to fully focus on Jesus.

God uses fasting to enlighten the eyes of your heart so you begin to perceive the presence of your exalted bridegroom. How much do you want to engage Him? Is it enough to try a biblically prescribed way to enhance your spiritual perception? Worship to come into His unseen presence. Fast to focus the eyes of your heart on the Lord.

Communion through His glory

You not only come to the Lord through worship but He

comes to you through His glory. God's glory is the shinning out of His manifest presence. 2 Corinthians 4:6 says,

> *"For God, who said, 'Let light shine out of darkness,' made his light shine in our hearts to give us the light of the knowledge of the glory of God in the face of Christ."*

The light of God's glory in Jesus comes with different degrees of brilliance.

Again, the scripture indicates that God comes in greater degrees of His glory through fasting. Moses, during a forty-day fast, was able to see the glory of God pass by as he was hidden in the cleft of a rock (Exodus 33:18–23). Daniel, after several weeks of fasting, testified that a powerful manifestation of glory came to him. It knocked him to the ground, caused him to lose his speech and shook him violently (Daniel 10:5–10). The one who Daniel saw looked very similar to the exalted Jesus John saw in his revelation (Revelation 1:12–16). Paul who writes that he fasted often also speaks of mighty revelations of the Lord (2 Corinthians 11:23–27; 12:2–4). One church father said that fasting to seek Jesus could be, "like a window full of light through which God looks, revealing himself to the intellect."[3]

Why does fasting increase the intensity of God's glory? It creates a greater capacity to receive in your human spirit. It is like opening the shutters to a window so that more sunlight comes in. How much more of God's glory could you experience if you would fast in faith for these manifestations of your absent bridegroom?

A taste of heaven

Guy Bevington lived a lifestyle of fasting. Once he

attempted to minister in a church but because of his uncompromising message the pastor asked him to leave the meeting and get out of town. Bevington had no transportation so he began to walk in a blizzard. As he traveled in the country away from the town he wondered where he would stay that night. The Lord spoke to him saying, "This is the place." To Bevington's surprise it was a huge haystack covered with snow. So he burrowed back into it some twelve feet and made a pillow out of his suitcase.

As he lay down Bevington said, "Well praise God, I don't reckon Jesus ever had it much better than this and probably most of the time not nearly as good." Suddenly the haystack lit up on the inside. Bevington said, "It was the most beautiful sight I ever saw. It looked like crystallized straw . . . forming a beautiful network." Bevington feared he had somehow caught the haystack on fire when he was crawling into it because of some matches in his pocket. But he said when he reached up and touched the straw it was cold and damp. He goes on to say, "Oh beloved, I will never be able this side of heaven to draw a worthy picture of the scene and also of the dazzling going on down in the soul. I have often thought that was a foretaste of what heaven is going to be." He reported that although the manifestation of glory lasted only a short time, there were raptures of exceedingly great joy that came in wave after wave as he lay in the splendor of this glory.

After this experience Bevington went back to the town he had left and spent eight more days in fasting and prayer. Revival hit the church with supernatural force. The pastor who had asked him to leave was eventually filled with the Holy Spirit. Guy Bevington concludes, "There is no doubt but that God would give us wonderful revelations if He could get us in condition to receive them."[4]

The Lord Jesus Christ longs to come to you in wonderful revelations of His glory if He could get you in condition to receive them. It might not light up a haystack but it can bring a "dazzling going on down in the soul." Fasting is one condition that opens you up to His glory. In Song of Songs 2:9 the young maiden says of her absent lover,

> *"My lover is like a gazelle, a young stag.*
> *Look! There he stands behind our wall,*
> *gazing through the window,*
> *peering through the lattice."*

Jesus, your absent lover, comes to you. His face peers through the lattice of this natural world. Fasting enlightens the eyes of your heart to perceive Him in passionate worship. It also opens up the window of your spirit to greater light, to streams "of the glory of God in the face of Christ." It was for this reason that Jesus said,

> *"The time will come when the bridegroom will be taken away from them, and on that day they will fast."*
> (Mark 2:20)

Notes

1. Zacharias Tanee Fomum, *The Ministry of Fasting* (Mumbai: Crossroads Communication, 1991) pp. 244–245
2. G.E.H. Palmer, Philip Sherrard and Kallistos Ware – translators, *The Philokalia* (Boston: Faber and Faber, 1984), Vol. 1, p. 259
3. Ibid, Vol. 3, p. 17
4. G.C. Bevington, *Remarkable Incidents and Modern Miracles through Prayer and Faith* (Kokomo: New Book Room) pp. 188–199

Chapter 10

The Door to Deliverance

"Your night will become like the noonday."
(Isaiah 58:10)

The Darkness of God's Wrath

Isaiah 58:10 describes a deliverance from darkness. Light from heaven drives away spiritual darkness when the door to deliverance is opened. One key that opens this door is fasting. Several causes for spiritual darkness exist. Fasting brings the noonday light of heaven into each of these areas.

There is the darkness of God's wrath. The wrath of God is not like human anger that seeks to destroy. His judgment comes out of compassion. God announces His judgment so that you will change. Divine wrath is a wake up call. If you will not listen to His words then listen to your pain. God sends the pain of judgment to wake you up from sin.

How do you come out of divine judgment? Jeremiah 18:7–8 says,

> *"If at any time I announce that a nation or kingdom is to be uprooted, torn down and destroyed, and if that nation*

I warned repents of its evil, then I will relent and not inflict the disaster I had planned."

Judgment is to get you to repent, not to wipe you out. Change your heart and it opens the way for God to change His. You change God's emotions through repentance.

Repent with fasting

Add fasting to repentance and it kicks into a different gear. Joel describes the signs of God's coming wrath. He also proclaims God's cry in the midst of the judgment.

> *"'Even now,' declares the LORD,*
> *'return to me with all your heart,*
> *with fasting and weeping and mourning.'"*
>
> (Joel 2:12)

Joel continues,

> *"Rend your heart*
> *and not your garments.*
> *Return to the LORD your God*
> *for he is gracious and compassionate,*
> *slow to anger and abounding in love*
> *and he relents from sending calamity."*
>
> (Joel 2:13)

Repentance delivers us from God's judgment. Add fasting to your repentance and it intensifies that repentance. When Jonah went to Nineveh he proclaimed that in forty days the city would be destroyed through God's wrath. To Jonah's surprise the people of the pagan city heard God's warning and repented. The King issued a decree to all the people. It said,

> *"Do not let any man or beast, herd or flock, taste anything; do not let them eat or drink. But let man and beast be covered with sackcloth. Let everyone call urgently on God. Let them give up their evil ways and their violence. Who knows? God may yet relent and with compassion turn from his fierce anger so that we will not perish."* (Jonah 3:7–9)

Notice that even the livestock fasted. Are you going to let the cows and sheep of Nineveh surpass you in your repentance and fasting? Jonah 3:10 reports,

> *"When God saw what they did and how they turned from their evil ways, he had compassion and did not bring upon them the destruction he had threatened."*

If you are in the night of God's wrath, seek the Lord with all your heart. Repent and fast before the Lord. Who knows? He may relent and with compassion turn from His judgment. Listen to the wake-up call. Don't turn it off and roll back over into your sin. Wake up with repentance and fasting!

The darkness of the demonic

There is another spiritual darkness. It is the darkness of demonic attack. Isaiah 49:24–25 says,

> *"Can plunder be taken from warriors*
> *or captives rescued from the fierce?*
> *But this is what the Lord says . . .*
> *'I will contend with those who contend with you,*
> *and your children I will save.'"*

Demonic spirits contend with you and your loved ones. God breaks their power through fasting.

One church father said,

> "Fast before the Lord according to your strength for to do this will purge you of your iniquities and sins; it exalts the soul, sanctifies the mind, drives away demons and prepares you for God's presence."[1]

Historically those who have a super-abundance of faith, particularly in the face of evil, spend much time in prayer and fasting.

Pastor Blumhardt of Germany had a deliverance ministry. He discovered the power of fasting and its effects upon the demonic. Experimenting with fasting, he spent thirty hours or more in fasting before a deliverance session. "I tried it [fasting], without telling anyone," he reported, "and in truth the later conflict was extraordinarily lightened by it. I could speak with much greater restfulness and decision. I did not require to be so long present with the sick one [demonized], and I felt I could influence without being present." He grew in effectiveness in his ministry over the demonic as he fasted.[2]

Pastor Hsi of China also became powerful in the area of deliverance. He brought hundreds of demonized people to freedom and many were healed under his ministry. He eventually took the name Sheng-Mo which means "conqueror of demons." After his conversion, his wife started manifesting demonically while seeking Christ. He called his household to a three-day fast. He claimed the promises of God. Pastor Hsi commanded the demons to leave his wife and stop their torment. She was instantly delivered and became a believer in Jesus Christ.[3]

In Mark 9:29 Jesus tells His disciples that certain demons can only come out by prayer and fasting.

Although some of the earliest manuscripts of the scripture do not have the word "fasting," Henry Gallus argues that even in these manuscripts it is implied since Jesus is speaking of praying with all your heart. Experience proves that it is true. Fasting shifts deliverance into a higher gear. When fasting and faith in the power of Jesus Christ are added to deliverance it springs people out of their demonic darkness.

The darkness of human sin

Finally, fast for deliverance from the darkness of human sin. You can fast concerning sin within your own life or evil within someone else's life. St. Isaac of Syria said,

> "The work of fasting and vigil is the beginning of every endeavor directed against sin and lust, especially in the case of a man who fights against the sin which is within. This practice shows hatred of sin and lust in the doer of this invisible warfare. Almost all passionate impulses decrease through fasting."[4]

Fasting is not an act of righteousness that cancels out sin. It is a way for God's grace to come through faith and win the battles over habitual sin. Fast for deliverance from sin.

Fasting can also bring deliverance from the sinful influence of another person. King Darius fasted for Daniel's deliverance from the lions' den. Some evil advisors and an unwise law put the King in a place where Daniel had to be executed. Daniel 6:18 says,

> *"Then the king returned to his palace and spent the night without eating and without entertainment being brought to him. And he could not sleep."*

The next morning after God delivered Daniel from the lions the King wrote a decree. He recognized that God alone had saved Daniel from the sinful influence of his advisors. The King praised God saying,

> *"He rescues and he saves;*
> *he performs signs and wonders*
> *in the heavens and on the earth.*
> *He has rescued Daniel*
> *from the power of the lions.* (Daniel 6:27)

Someone clearly summarized this story. Because the King fasted the lions fasted as well!

Deliverance from family chaos

God introduced me to fasting during a critical time in our family. We were unraveling because of difficulties one of our children was experiencing as a teenager. I started fasting. God began to move. After one fast God revealed to me that I was not taking seriously the cries of my son. I had to be delivered from my own sins before my son could be. God helped my wife and me make some hard and difficult decisions for our son that previously I wasn't willing to make.

In the midst of the turbulence God gave us unusual seasons of peace when we needed them. Whenever I fasted there was a breakthrough. It wasn't always dramatic but it was significant. Toward the end of our son's struggles, I was in a long fast when he called from a Youth With A Mission base in Australia. He shared how he had been filled with the Spirit. The power of God knocked him down twice. His experience made me hungry for a greater expression of the Spirit's work in my own life.

There are many factors which can bring healing and

deliverance into our families. I'm convinced fasting is an important way in which God's light scatters the darkness. His light may not be at noonday, but it sure is climbing higher in the sky. The son I used to fast for now fasts for me. Fasting brings deliverance from the shadow of God's wrath, the night of demonic bondage and the fog of human sin. Fast for the sunrise of God's transforming light.

Notes

1. G.E.H. Palmer, Philip Sherrard and Kallistos Ware – translators, *The Philokalia* (Boston: Faber and Faber, 1984), Vol. 1, p. 36
2. Arthur Wallis, *God's Chosen Fast* (Pennsylvania: Christian Literature Crusade, 1968) p. 68
3. Ibid, p. 67
4. E. Kadloubovsky and G.E.H. Palmer – translators, *Writings from the Philokalia on Prayer of the Heart* (Boston: Faber and Faber, 1951) p. 206

Chapter 11

The Door to Guidance

"The LORD *will guide you always."*
(Isaiah 58:11)

Back to the Future

How important is divine guidance? It is not very important if you see yourself facing your future. As you walk confidently into your future you might need the Lord's help on a few hard decisions. But since you can see most of what is coming toward you, God's help is not all that important. The problem with this view of life, however, is that it is wrong. The truth is you face the past, not the future. You know where you have been but you don't know where you are going! You don't march into the future. You back into it. God, however, always faces the future even as you face the past. He sees everything the future holds and can navigate you through it. Do you want to enter into God's future? As you face the past, reach behind in faith, let Him grip your hand and lead you into your purpose.[1]

Most people back into the future without God. But if you are to find God's purpose for you, divine guidance is essential. Romans 8:14 says,

> *"Those who are led by the Spirit of God are sons of God."*

When you become a child of God, He grips your spirit with His Holy Spirit so He can guide your steps. Fasting makes your spirit more sensitive to the Holy Spirit's grip. His guidance then becomes clear and continual. Isaiah explains that after you fast, *"the Lord will guide you always."* Divine guidance comes in different ways. Fasting can enhance your perception of God's direction in each of these areas. Move into your destiny by keeping tender to the guidance of the Lord.

The gentle pressure of the Holy Spirit

God guides you by His touch. Divine touch is the Spirit's gentle and constant pressure upon your spirit which confirms you are going in God's direction. Romans 8:16 says,

> *"The Spirit himself testifies with our spirit that we are God's children."*

He also testifies to your spirit by His peaceful touch that you are tracking with God's purpose. You can guide a child without a word. The gentle pull of your hand directs her. Your touch on her shoulder guides her. In the same way, the Holy Spirit's pressure of peace on your spirit is the primary means of daily guidance.

But other pressures can distract you from the Holy Spirit's touch. At times, very turbulent circumstances can disorient you from God's purpose. The outward pressures of suffering and spiritual warfare eclipse your ability to feel the Lord's gentle touch. Even success and popularity can distract you from the touch of the Holy Spirit. The strong pressure of self-fulfillment entices you away from God's guidance on your life. Stay sensitive to the Holy Spirit's touch in both difficult and enjoyable circumstances. One way to strengthen your tenderness to the Spirit's touch is fasting.

Nehemiah fasted for the returning exiles of Jerusalem. A benefit of that fast was greater sensitivity to God's guidance. Nehemiah needed guidance in the rebuilding of the walls because he faced many difficult experiences. Since he was tender to God's touch he navigated through all the difficulties to arrive at God's purpose (Nehemiah 1:3–4).

David Brainerd fasted. He too had to know God's guiding touch. Only then could he bring the American Indians to Christ through some extremely difficult experiences. He wrote,

> "Set apart this day for fasting and prayer to God for His grace, especially to prepare me for the work of ministry; to give me divine aid and direction in my preparations for the great work and in His own time to send me into His harvest."[2]

Whether you face dark difficulties or stunning successes you must have a sense of the Spirit's touch that transcends all of these experiences. Fast for a greater tenderness to the Holy Spirit's pressure on your spirit.

The authority of His Word

The Holy Spirit not only guides you by His touch but also by His Word. When God speaks it is an authoritative word. He guides you by the pressure of His peace through His touch. He also guides you by the authority of His voice through His Word. Jesus said,

> *"But when he, the Spirit of truth, comes, he will guide you into all truth. He will not speak on his own; he will*

> *speak only what he hears, and he will tell you what is yet to come."* (John 16:13)

The Spirit speaks to you in several ways. He guides you through the Scriptures. You don't have to seek guidance when the Scriptures have already shown you what to do. In that case follow the lead of the Spirit through His inspired written Word. Read the Bible to know what He is saying. Then do it. At times the Spirit will speak to you with a portion of the Scriptures that becomes the guiding truth for your life.

The Holy Spirit also guides you by His inward voice. Paul asks,

> *"Don't you know that you yourselves are God's temple and that God's Spirit lives in you?"*
> (1 Corinthians 3:16)

The indwelling Holy Spirit speaks directly into your spirit to guide. This inward voice must always be in agreement with the written Word of God. The Holy Spirit guides through His voice deep in your spirit. Again, you can increase your sensitivity to the voice of the Holy Spirit by fasting. In Acts 13:2 the leaders of the church in Antioch are fasting when the Holy Spirit says,

> *"Set apart for me Barnabas and Saul for the work to which I have called them."*

How did the Spirit's voice come to these men? It must have been an inner voice of guidance spoken out by someone through prophecy. Notice God had already called Paul and Barnabas to a work. Possibly the leaders fasted to get direction about God's previous call. Their guidance, which came through prophecy, was for confirmation.

The first forty-day fast I ever did was to pray for protection against an attack upon our family. I was convinced everything would be wonderful after the fast. Instead it became worse! But in the midst of the difficulties I could clearly hear the voice of the Lord. He gave me a divine strategy and a powerful promise for getting through this very difficult time. Now I realize the forty-day fast was not for protection from our problem. It was for hearing the voice of God. If you can hear from your Commander in the midst of the battle, eventually He will lead you to victory.

Fast to hear the voice of the Holy Spirit. Listen to Him through the reading of the Word or the confirming guidance of His inner voice.

Spectacular guidance

The Holy Spirit guides through His touch, His voice and His signs. Signs are the more spectacular expression of guidance. Through a dream, a vision or an angelic visitation the Spirit gives a sign that clearly shows the way. Because guidance through a sign is so dramatic you can be enamored by it as the only way God guides. God does use spectacular means but it is not His common way of guidance. It wasn't in the New Testament and it isn't today. Usually He guides through His touch of peace and through His voice, particularly through His voice in the Bible.

God reserves signs for the more difficult cases. For example, He had to get Peter, a Jew, to share the gospel in the house of Cornelius, a Gentile. Every cell in Peter's body was repulsed by such a notion. From his first day of understanding he was taught that Gentiles were unclean. To make contact with them was a sin. So God pulled out the stops. The first sign God sent was an angelic visitation to Cornelius so he would have the courage to invite a Jew to his Gentile home. Second, God gave Peter the sign of an open vision repeated three times. He was re-educating Peter not to call anything impure that God had made clean, including Gentiles. Third, the Holy Spirit spoke to Peter with a clear sign. It was a word of knowledge and direction to go to Cornelius' house. Finally, God poured out a stunning manifestation of the Holy Spirit on Cornelius' household as a sign that the conversion of the Gentiles was God's will (Acts 10:1–48).

Don't pursue signs over the more common means of guidance simply because signs are more exciting. But you can seek signs in very difficult situations. Fasting opens heaven for this unusual means of guidance to come. Dreams, visions and angelic visitations about Jesus in the Muslim and Hindu world have increased as Christians fast and pray for the 10/40 Window. This is clear evidence that fasting and prayer can bring signs to closed people groups.

During an enforced fast because of a storm at sea, Paul had an important angelic visitation. The visitation was critical for Paul to convince the Romans not to execute him or any of the other prisoners on the sinking ship (Acts 27:21–26). Signs are not the norm. But there are critical times when God sends signs. Fasting opens the way for these unusual manifestations of guidance to come.

Guidance to salvation

Steve, whom I mentioned in the introduction of the book, attended Bible College in Canberra, Australia. One week the Principal informed the students and the faculty that classes were cancelled to have a week long fast in the school chapel. Steve reported that those days of fasting were a highlight in his spiritual life.

After a week of fasting, Steve went to his room to rest. Lying on his bed he suddenly had a vision of a man in an alley on a motorcycle. Steve recognized the alley as one in downtown Canberra. The Spirit said to Steve, "Go there immediately." Steve borrowed the Principal's car and went downtown. There in the alley was the man on the cycle just as Steve saw it in his vision. The man was surprised to see Steve at that late hour. Steve simply said, "The Lord has sent me to you." The man broke down weeping. When he got his composure he shared with Steve that he had prayed earlier to God, "If you don't do something, I'm going to kill myself." Steve led him and eventually his family to the Lord. A week of fasting opened Steve's spirit to a spectacular sign from God's compassionate heart.

Seek direction for your life or for someone else's life. Fast for an environment where God guides. After a good fast *"the LORD will guide you always"* (Isaiah 58:11).

Notes

1. Taken from a message by Dr Dennis Kinlaw dealing with the Hebrew concept of the future, present and past.
2. David Smith, *Fasting A Neglected Discipline* (Chichester: New Wine Press, 1954) p. 55

Chapter 12

The Door to Provision

"The Lord . . . will satisfy your needs
in a sun-scorched land."
(Isaiah 58:11)

Provision or Prosperity

Provision is one benefit of fasting. Isaiah says that when there is nothing, the Lord will provide as you fast before Him. Do you pull back from the idea of provision from God? One reason you may have a negative reaction is that you confuse provision with the recent prosperity teaching. But there is a world of difference between prosperity and provision.

One prosperity teacher told how he believed God for a car that cost a hundred and twenty five thousand dollars. It was a Rolls Royce. He then quoted the words of Jesus, *"What things so ever you desire."* He confessed that he desired that kind of car. He said, "Some people like dogs and some people like cats and I wanted a Rolls Royce." So he believed God for it. He proclaimed that it is your faith that gets you what you want. That is prosperity teaching.[1]

Provision is different. The Pilgrims experienced a great drought that lasted from the end of May until the middle of July. It threatened their entire corn crop. The Pilgrims set aside a day of prayer and fasting. God answered so quickly that it amazed not only the Pilgrims but also the Native-Americans who witnessed God's generous response. A gentle, continuous rain came. It fully soaked the ground and produced a bountiful crop of corn.[2]

What is the difference between prosperity and provision? Prosperity is an aggressive faith for what you want. Provision is believing God for what you need. God promises to satisfy your needs in a sun-scorched land. Isaiah doesn't say God will satisfy your wants in a materially glutted society. He will give you what you need. Fasting is the key to open the door to provision.

The Hebrew prophet, Joel, tells of God's provision through fasting. He describes the conditions necessary to fast for provision. God wants to meet your needs through fasting. Look at how Joel says it happens.

Poor, blind and naked

The first condition for the provision of God is to discover your need. If provision is God meeting your need, you must first know your need. It wasn't hard for the people of Judah to see their need. Joel describes a people who mourn, languish and lament (Joel 1). The Jews reacted this way because wave after wave of locusts had come upon the land, devastating their crops. Next, a scorching drought burned up everything that the locusts left behind. Desolation is how Joel described the land. It was so bad that no one could remember it ever being that bad. There wasn't even enough grain or wine to carry on the sacrifices to bless the Lord. It was a "sun-scorched land."

More than likely you don't have any great needs like that. Yours is a good life with more food and stuff than you can handle. You certainly don't live in a sun-scorched land. But Revelation 3:17 declares,

> *"You say, 'I am rich; I have acquired wealth and do not need a thing.' But you do not realize that you are wretched, pitiful, poor, blind and naked."*

In other words, there is more than one kind of sun-scorched land. If you live in this prosperous nation you are still in need. There has been an invasion of demonic locusts that have stripped you of vibrant faith in God, power to minister and a life committed to the Gospel's expansion. Lament, quake and mourn for our condition! The church is drying up. Has this nation ever seen a spiritual drought like this? There is not even enough offering of faith to please the Lord.

If you don't see our need it is because you don't see what God wants. God is not looking for a Church that simply survives the present cultural chaos. He doesn't want a Church that looks back on some past achievements of faith. God wants a people who are transforming their communities. He wants a Church that launches out hundreds of believers into ministry. He wants you filled with His fire of holiness.

Are you convinced it is impossible? You can't imagine how you can live the way God wants you to live in this selfish society. How can you possibly have spiritual power in this sin-scorched culture? That is the point. You can't. Instead, believe God for His provision to get you there. God wants to do something in you that is impossible for this generation. There is no way we as the Church can get to where God wants us. And that's not a bad place to be. It means we have a need so big that only God can meet it through His provision.

See. You do have a need in a sun-scorched culture. That fulfills the first condition to fast for provision.

Aggressive faith or brokenness

Second, when you fast for provision, link your fasting to brokenness. Humble yourself. Again in Joel you find that fasting is coupled with weeping, turning and repenting (Joel 2:12–17). Joel 2:13 speaks of "rending your heart." That is brokenness. Remember how fasting is a way of shifting other spiritual realities into a higher gear? Fasting intensifies prayer, worship and deliverance. It also intensifies brokenness. That's important because brokenness is the key to God's provision.

The Pilgrims spoke of fasting as humiliation. It was a way for them to humble themselves. God also ordained one day a year for the Jews to afflict their souls, the Day of Atonement. This affliction meant they were to humble themselves through fasting. Don't stand in the way of God meeting your need by wildly running around to solve all your problems. Repent of such arrogance. Fast to recognize that you can't meet your need. This is another difference between prosperity and provision. Prosperity is an aggressive faith where you go full throttle after what you want. Provision is humbling yourself before the Lord to believe Him for what you need. Prosperity comes through desire-asserting faith. Provision comes through a self-humbling faith. Fasting intensifies this brokenness. The people of Judah humbled themselves with fasting in the book of Joel. Hannah, in 1 Samuel 1, humbled herself with a fast, weeping and broken for God's provision of a son.

On April 30, 1863 Abraham Lincoln, in the middle of a civil war that was tearing the United States apart, proclaimed a national day of fasting, prayer and humiliation. Lincoln explained,

> "Intoxicated with unbroken success, we have become too self-sufficient to feel the necessity of redeeming and preserving grace, too proud to pray to God that made us! It behooves us, then to humble ourselves before the offended Power, to confess our sins and to pray for clemency and forgiveness."[3]

The Spirit of God comes with provision when all barriers of self-importance, self-sufficiency and arrogance are brought low. The provision of God comes on the tracks of brokenness and humility. Fasting helps you lay those tracks.

Abundant provision

When you fast for provision, prepare to be surprised by God's abundance. Joel speaks of provisions that are plenteous, satisfying and overflowing (Joel 2:19–32). The picture of God's provision in Joel 2:28 is of a vessel being poured out. This is the great prophecy about the outpouring of the Holy Spirit which became the text for Peter's Pentecost sermon. Now, that is satisfaction!

Isaiah 58 proclaims that your needs will be satisfied. But understand that God's provision is so extravagant that He will satisfy more than your needs. His provision will splash over and satisfy the needs of others. Look at Hannah. Yes, she got her son, Samuel, but she also got a provision that blessed an entire nation. She didn't just get her baby, she got a prophet for Israel. God's provision is abundant (1 Samuel 1:24–28). Not only will God satisfy you and others, He will also satisfy Himself. Remember in Joel that Judah didn't have enough grain to worship God. But the Lord said He would send enough so that,

> *"You will have plenty to eat, until you are full,*

> *and you will praise the name of the Lord your God,*
> *who has worked wonders."* (Joel 2:26)

God will be satisfied with the praises of His people. His outpouring of provision splashes back to Him.

Miraculous provision

When Youth With A Mission was preparing the first ministry ship to be launched in Greece, 175 young people were finishing a forty-day corporate fast. One of the ship's crew was walking along the beach when twelve medium-sized fish jumped out of a shallow pool. The young missionaries celebrated with a fish fry that night. It was a welcome break from the rice they had been eating when they were not fasting. A few days later a large tuna jumped out of the sea. They again feasted on fish. Then one of the team members was praying near the ocean and suddenly fish began to jump out of the water all over the beach. She got the attention of some local Greek families. They came down to help her gather the fish. The young girl gathered 210 fish and the neighbors gathered two to three times more. The next Tuesday at 8 AM the fish started jumping again. The mission team got containers and started collecting the fish. The amazed Greeks exclaimed, "God is with this people." That morning the Greek neighbors and the youth collected over one ton of fish. It was a time of praise and feasting.[4]

God was saying, "I will supply your need." It was like the miraculous catch of fish when Jesus told Peter to launch out into the deep. After the catch, Jesus called Peter to be a fisher of men (Luke 5:1–11). God gave these fasting young people a prophetic provision as well. It spoke of the countless people that would be brought into the kingdom through the ministry of the YWAM ships.

When you fast God doesn't just provide. He lavishes His provision on you.

Notes

1. Frederick K.C. Price, *How Faith Works* (Tulsa: Harrison House, 1996) p. 247
2. Derek Prince, *Shaping History Through Prayer and Fasting* (Fort Lauderdale: Derek Prince Ministries, 1973) p. 136
3. Prince, ibid, pp.6–7
4. Loren Cunningham, *Is That Really You, God?* (Seattle: YWAM Publishing, 1984) pp. 149–150

Chapter 13

The Door to Anointing

"You will be like a well-watered garden,
like a spring whose waters never fail."
(Isaiah 58:11)

White Water Flow

Once, the Lord gave me a vision of a cave with a body of still water. The water was so clear I could see the shapes and colors under its surface. The Lord revealed that the water represented His Holy Spirit in me. The vision was beautiful. He then informed me that even though it was beautiful it wasn't all He wanted. Next, the Lord showed me the same scene in the cave but this time the water wasn't still, instead it was flowing turbulently with white water splashing off the sides. He whispered to me, "Mark, in you I want My Spirit to flow." The anointing of God comes from the flow of the Spirit. Jesus said,

> *"Whoever believes in me . . . streams of living water will flow from within him."* (John 7:38)

John goes on to comment,

> *"By this he meant the Spirit."* (John 7:39)

How do you see this white water flow of the Spirit fulfilled? Many factors contribute to the flow of the Holy Spirit. But one of the means for a greater flow is fasting. Isaiah 58:11 says if you give yourself to a fasting lifestyle you will be like *"a spring whose waters never fail."* Spiritual fruit is produced because the Spirit constantly flows out of you.

John Lake saw thousands of people radically healed through his ministry. Where did he get such a flow of power? He testified,

> "I went into fasting and prayer and waiting on God for nine months. And one day, the glory of God in a new manifestation and a new incoming came to my life ... God flowed through me with a new force. Healings were of a more powerful order. Oh, God lived in me, God manifested in me, God spoke through me."[1]

Jesus also demonstrated this truth. It wasn't enough for Jesus to receive the Holy Spirit for a fruitful ministry. After He had received the baptism of the Holy Spirit He entered a forty-day fast. One result of that fast was an increase of the Spirit's flow. Look at what this same flow of the Spirit can manifest through your life.

Astonishing authority

Authority is manifest in you through the flow of the Holy Spirit. Anointed truth has authority. After Jesus' forty-day fast the response to His teaching was astonishment. In Capernaum the people *"were amazed at his teaching, because his message had authority."* In Nazareth they *"were amazed at the gracious words that came from his lips"* (Luke 4:32, 22). Jesus hotly pursued the truth of God. Satan tried to distort the truth of Scriptures in the wilderness. He tempted Jesus with lies to dam up the flow of God's truth. But Jesus overcame the deception of the enemy by knowing the truth and obeying it. Jesus used His time of fasting to both get into the truth and get the truth in Him. When He went out to minister the Word, it was clear, passionate and without compromise.

One way to see divine authority in you is to know God's Word. If you want to bring that authority to a white water flow then fast your way into God's truth. When the truth flows through you in the anointing of the Holy Spirit there will be authority.

Savanarola came to Florence in 1491. His ministry exploded in power and affected the entire community. Because he preached truth with authority, revival broke out in the city. Savanarola's uncompromising preaching eventually cost him his life. What was the secret to his authority? He would fast, seeking God day and night until he discovered his message in the truth of the Scriptures. Often Savanarola was so weak from fasting before preaching that he needed help to remain in the pulpit. James Burns, describing the white water flow of Savanarola's authority, writes,

> "The sentences rushed out, never halting, never losing intensity or volume, but growing until his voice became as the voice of God Himself, and all the building rocked and swayed as if it moved to the mighty passion of his words."[2]

Look at the reformers and revivalists who proclaimed truth with authority. They not only knew God's Word but they fasted their way into the truth. Martin Luther,

John Knox, John Wesley and Charles Finney all fasted and prayed. Jonathan Edwards preached with such authority that revival came to New England. Why did he see revival? He knew the Word of God but there was more. He fasted. He not only fasted but he fasted so often it was sometimes hard for him to maintain his balance while standing to preach.

The white water flow of the Spirit manifests in you through authority. Know the truth of God's Word. Fast into that truth. Then minister it in the anointing of His divine authority.

When God comes

God's presence is also manifested in you through the flow of the Holy Spirit. When Jesus came into a setting there was an incredible sense of the presence of God. Demons would manifest calling Jesus the "Holy One of God." Peter fell at Jesus' feet and was convicted of his sinfulness. Crowds gathered because of the sense of God's presence in Jesus. Jesus made the manifest presence of God the heart of His message. He proclaimed that in His coming the kingdom of God was near (Luke 4:34; 5:8, 19; Mark 1:15).

During His time in the wilderness Jesus refused the temptations of the enemy by giving himself fully to God. He also fasted into the presence of His Father. Even His cousin, John, had learned this truth. John was absolutely committed to the will of God. He too fasted into God's presence through a partial fast of locust and honey. The presence of God manifested so strongly in John that within a six-month period revival shook the region through his ministry. People from all levels of society and from all over the country traveled out to the desert to experience his ministry. Through this very ministry the Spirit fell in power upon Jesus (Luke 4:6–8; Mark 1:5–10).

The presence of God can be manifest in you through the flow of the Holy Spirit. Give yourself fully to God. Then fast into His presence. This is one means by which the anointing can increase to a white water flow.

Gwen Shaw had been a missionary for fourteen years but there was a lack of God's anointing on her ministry. One day God sent a man to minister at her church in China. Through this man she saw people experience the transforming presence of God. Gwen said, "I saw God do more through His anointed servant in fourteen days than I had been able to do in fourteen years." After she witnessed the presence and love of God in this minister she asked, "Brother, what is the secret of God's anointing in your life?" He answered, "There are two things I have done which many of God's workers never have done – I have given myself to God one hundred percent, and I have fasted." His answer led to Gwen's first fast. During that fast God spoke to her of the importance of giving herself fully to Him. The Lord said, "You think you know consecration, but that which you have consecrated is nothing in comparison to this complete yielding up of *all*. I want you to die – so you might live an abundant life."[3] This fast took Gwen into a season that brought the presence of God into her ministry like she had never known.

Die to your self-interests. Give yourself totally to God in obedience to His will. Then fast into His presence and believe that the velocity of God's anointing will increase to become a white water flow.

The day of His power

Another characteristic of the flow of the Holy Spirit is power. When Jesus experienced His Spirit baptism, Luke 4:1 says,

> *"Jesus, full of the Holy Spirit, returned from the Jordan."*

After the forty-day fast Jesus took a passage from Isaiah at the Nazareth synagogue. He believed the Spirit of the Lord was on Him to do the anointed ministry of the kingdom (Luke 4:16–21). Then in rapid-fire succession He started to do that ministry. He healed the sick, delivered the demonized, saved the lost and empowered His disciples.

After His baptism He was filled with the Holy Spirit but after His fast the white water flow of the Spirit's power was released. He believed and fasted into the power of the Spirit. At the end of the forty-day fast the Spirit who filled Jesus at the Jordan was now flowing out in spiritual turbulence. Luke reported,

> *"Jesus returned to Galilee in the power of the Spirit."* (Luke 4:14)

Later Luke wrote of this anointing,

> *"And the power of the Lord was present for him to heal the sick."* (Luke 5:17)

How do you enter into the power of the Holy Spirit? Get filled. Believe you can do the anointed works of the kingdom. Then do them. Jesus promised that streams of the Holy Spirit's power will flow out of you. Believe the promise by doing His works. As you do them remember that fasting in faith is one way to increase the flow of God's power.

I remember a testimony from Paul Bruton of the East African Mission. He told about a teenage African named Edwin who wanted papers to preach. Since he was uneducated the church said it would take twelve years of school for him to be approved. He came to Paul and explained, "There is a fire in me. I've got to preach. Do you have a paper I can use to preach?" Paul opened his Bible to Mark 16, read it and said, "Here is your authority." He took Edwin to a nearby town, set up a platform and got a crowd of one thousand two hundred people to hear him preach. Edwin announced to the crowd, "God has sent me here. I've been fasting and praying for a week. And God spoke to me. He said, 'In your first service I am going to perform a miracle so the people will know you are a man of God who has come with the message of God to do the work of God.'" Paul said he was listening to Edwin from his Land Rover. Fearing that Edwin had overstated God's intentions, Paul hid six inches below the steering wheel.

Edwin then said, "You don't know any songs I want to sing nor the service I want to follow, so let's just have the miracle now." He then stood and began to pray. When he finished his prayer he said, "Who has been healed?" Immediately a boy with one of his legs eight inches shorter than the other jumped off the hood of a car where he had been sitting. In the twenty feet between the car and the platform his leg grew eight inches. He began to shout, "It's me! It's me! I have been healed!" Edwin said, "I have come to tell you about Jesus and if He can heal a leg like this wouldn't you like to give your life to Him?" Three hundred and seventeen people came to receive Jesus that night.

Edwin is no exception. You too can experience the flow of the Holy Spirit's power. Believe for the works of Jesus. Do the works. Increase the flow of anointing through fasting.

Let the river flow

When my family and I first moved to Monterrey, Mexico, I noticed a map of the city. According to the map there was a large river flowing through the middle of Monterrey. When we arrived, however, there was no river. There was only a riverbed. The river had dried up years ago. The people of the city had transformed the riverbed into a string of soccer fields for recreation. Often, as I drove past the riverbed, I would see dust coming up as countless games of soccer were being played in the dried-up riverbed.

A riverbed works great as a soccer field but a riverbed is made for a river. Jesus said in the map of every believer's life there is a mighty river of His Spirit flowing in supernatural force. Unfortunately, many believers only have a riverbed. There is no flow of the Holy Spirit through their lives.

If you only have a riverbed, don't fill it up with frantic religious activity. It simply stirs up a lot of dust. God intends for your riverbed to be filled with the white water flow of His Holy Spirit. Jesus promised it to you. Know God's truth, give yourself wholly to God and do the works of Jesus. Fast in faith and watch the flow of divine anointing increase.

Notes

1. Roberts Liardon – compiler, *John G. Lake The Complete Collection of His Life Teachings* (Tulsa: Albury Publishing, 1999) p. 372
2. James Burns, *Revivals Their Laws and Leaders* (Grand Rapids: Baker, 1960) p. 139
3. Gwen Shaw, *Your Appointment With God* (Jasper: End-Time Handmaidens, Inc., 1977) pp. iiiv

Chapter 14

The Door to Revival

"Your people will rebuild the ancient ruins
and will raise up the age-old foundations."
(Isaiah 58:12)

Spiritual Ghost Towns

William Duma, a Zulu in South Africa, became the pastor of a dying church. He entered a twenty-one-day fast for his church. On the last day of the fast the glory of the Lord physically descended on him. God spoke to Duma, saying

> "My servant, you saw the tall cluster of white lilies growing so vigorously in the valley below: in just the same way your dead church will become a witness to me. You will see humanity transformed from darkness to light."[1]

When he returned to his church the demonized people cried out. He saw powerful signs of God's healing and delivering power. Hundreds came to the Lord. As he called his church to fast and pray each week, they experienced ongoing revival and healing.

Isaiah describes ancient ruins, age-old foundations,

broken walls and destroyed streets with empty dwellings (Isaiah 58:12). Here is a place, like Duma's church before his fast, that once held life but now it is a ghost town, completely fallen apart. Churches become ghost towns. Their spiritual life can disintegrate even when their facilities, programs and attendance don't. A church can be no more than the fossil from a previous move of God. Like a seashell, it is the beautiful remains of what once held life. For this reason revival is essential. Revival is when a church comes to life again or remains alive. Revival rebuilds, renews and repairs churches. Fasting is a key for the revival that transforms a church from a ghost town into a Holy Ghost assembly. Fasting can bring renewal to your church if you fast for these realities and believe for revival.

The DNA of church

Fast for church life. What is church life? It is supernatural life released into the people of God. Church life is the difference between a social group of believers and the body of Christ. Paul and Barnabas appointed elders from among the disciples in the region of Antioch. They prayed and fasted for them, committing them to the Lord. During that time a new level of church life came to the group (Acts 14:21–23).

The church is more than the accumulation of human presence, even Christian human presence. It is supernatural life flowing through a congregation of believers. Church life does not come through programs and techniques. It comes from heaven. Derek Prince, commenting on the above account of fasting from Acts, concludes,

> "It is therefore fair to say that the establishment of a local church in a city was accomplished by collective prayer and fasting."[2]

The International Charismatic Mission in Bogotá, one of the largest cell churches in the world, calls its members to fast and pray over the establishment of new cells. They recognize that if a cell is going to survive and multiply, it will happen because supernatural life is flowing. Divine life is the DNA for each cell. They fast because their life depends on it.

Church life is just as much a work of grace as Christian life. God's life came to you as a believer and it comes to you corporately as the people of God. The Church is a miracle born out of supernatural life in Christ Jesus. In Zechariah 4:6 God says, it is *"not by might, nor by power, but by my Spirit."* Then God illustrates this truth with a vision. The vision shows a lampstand connected into two pipes. The pipes supply golden oil to fuel the fire burning in the lampstand. The oil comes from two olive trees that feed into the pipes. Do you see it? The fuel to keep the church bright with supernatural life comes from a living source outside the church. It comes from the supernatural world. Fasting helps feed the flow of supernatural life into the church.

The Lord spoke to Mahesh Chavda and his wife, Bonnie, about calling their church to a twenty-one-day fast. The people were to pray together at 5:00 AM for two hours each morning. But only a handful of people showed up the first two mornings. At the mid-week evening service one man gave a prophetic word. He said, "The Lord told me, 'I am here, where are my people?' " Over the next few nights children started waking up and telling their parents to go to the church for the prayer meeting. The people came out and started fasting. The crowd eventually swelled to two hundred people. A revival of divine life rushed into the church lasting for weeks and transforming many people.[3]

How much do you want supernatural life to flow into your church? Fast and pray for church life.

After you fast

Fast for supernatural power. Divine power comes through the outpouring of the Holy Spirit. Joel says,

> *"And afterwards,*
> *I will pour out my Spirit on all people . . .*
> *Even on my servants, both men and women,*
> *I will pour out my Spirit in those days."*
>
> (Joel 2:28–29)

This was the passage Peter used to describe what happened when the Holy Spirit came in power at Pentecost (Acts 2:17–21). Peter went on to explain that this outpouring was not a unique event but was the common event of the last days. Since you live in the last days the outpouring of the Holy Spirit is also a promise for your church. Peter declares,

> *"The promise is for you and your children and for all who are far off – for all whom the Lord our God will call."*
>
> (Acts 2:39)

How can you experience such an outpouring of the Spirit? Joel shows one way this can happen. He says the Spirit will be poured out "after." But here's the question: after what? Three times prior to this verse Joel tells us what must be done before this outpouring of the Spirit comes. In three different places he calls the people to fast (Joel 1:14; 2:12, 15). The Spirit is poured out after fasting.

John Wesley reports in his journal about a group of Methodist believers showing very little life. They committed to fast every week. After the first week of fasting Wesley said, "God broke in upon them in a wonderful manner; His work has increased ever since.

The neighboring societies heard about what happened and agreed to follow the same rule: soon they experienced the same blessing." Wesley concludes his entry,

> "To neglect this specific duty (I mean fasting, ranked by our Lord with almsgiving and prayer) is one reason for deadness among Christians. Can anyone willingly neglect it without guilt?"[4]

Wesley asks a good question. This key unlocks the life-giving flow of the Holy Spirit upon the people of God. If there is deadness in your church, are you ignoring the key?

An open heaven opens hearts

Finally, fast for an open heaven. Fast that God will be so clearly present that even the world will know it. Once people experience an open heaven they can't stay away.

In Zechariah 8:18–20 God speaks of fasts that will become *"joyful and glad occasions and happy festivals."* Why will fasting bring such joy? God explains,

> *"In those days ten men from all languages and nations will take firm hold of one Jew by the hem of his robe and say, 'Let us go with you, because we have heard that God is with you.'"* (Zechariah 8:23)

Because of an open heaven Zechariah says that the people of God are revived. But it doesn't stop there. Revival will come to other cities. Nations will be drawn to the presence of God. The open heaven will be a magnet even to those who don't know the Lord (Zechariah 8:20–23).

In 1970 I experienced a spontaneous revival on the campus of Asbury College. It was interesting to watch how even the secular press was pulled into the revival because of the open heaven over the auditorium where we met. They came just to report on the unusual event. Some couldn't leave because God was with us. Students commented that the open heaven was like a divine magnet pulling people in and holding them in a loving atmosphere. Fast for an open heaven over your church.

Use the key

Without revival a church will dry up and wither. Revival is essential. This kingdom treasure is locked up in the storehouse of heaven. But God is not reluctant to send revival to His church. He desires that every church experience church life, supernatural power and an open heaven. He gives you the key that unlocks the door to revival.

Daniel Baker of Savannah, Georgia, in 1828 would regularly give a day to fasting and prayer. A tomb in a black cemetery became his place to seek the Lord. Through his use of the fasting key his congregation was revived and his ministry transformed. Until his death in 1857 he saw a continuous move of God with hundreds of new converts.[5]

How much do you want revival? Savanarola wanted revival so much that many times he had to be helped to stand and preach. He was so weak from using this key. But he unlocked the door for a mighty transformation of Florence. Wesley so desired revival that he told those who wanted to be Methodist preachers to fast at least twice a week. Otherwise they need not join him. With the fasting key they did something few people have done in church history. They maintained the flow of revival for over fifty years. Whenever Charles Finney saw the power of revival diminishing in his ministry he used the key. "The power would return on me," he said, "with all freshness." He wanted revival so much that he fasted to change a nation.

God gives you the key that unlocks the door to one of the great treasures of His kingdom. Are you ready to take it up, put it in the lock and turn it? Fast for revival!

Notes

1. Mary Garnett, *Take Your Glory Lord* (Kent: Sovereign World, 2000) pp. 26, 27
2. Derek Prince, *Shaping History Through Prayer and Fasting* (Fort Lauderdale: Derek Prince Ministries, 1973) p. 84
3. Mahesh Chavda, *The Hidden Power of Prayer and Fasting* (Shippensburg: Destiny Image, 1998) pp. 94–96
4. Nehemiah Curnock (ed.), *The Journal of the Rev. John Wesley, A.M.* (London: The Epworth Press, 1938) Vol. 5, p. 17
5. Brian H. Edwards, *Revival!* (Durham: Evangelical Press, 1990) p. 76

Chapter 15

The Worn Key

"Only a day for a man to humble himself?"
(Isaiah 58:5)

A Fasting Lifestyle

As I look at the keys on my key ring I find some are worn through constant use. Others are sharp and shiny because I rarely use them. The keys that are well-used open doors to places I regularly go. Fasting needs to be a worn key. Fasting is not meant to be a one-time event. Maybe you have done a forty-day fast and that's all. Or you occasionally use fasting when a crisis comes up. It is a key that is rarely used or even remembered.

Although fasting has merit as an occasional event, its greatest blessing is when you regularly use it. Fasting is not just an event. It is a lifestyle. You can develop this lifestyle in a safe and enjoyable way. Here are some tips to help you adjust physically, mentally and spiritually for many fasts in the coming years.

Wade in and go slow

Make your fast physically sound. If you have never fasted, wade slowly into the lifestyle. For your first fast don't plunge into forty days unless the Lord calls you to do it. Instead, seek the Lord for a gradual entrance into fasting. Give your body time to adjust. Begin by fasting a meal. Move the next week to fast for a day. After several weeks do a three-day fast. Usually after three days of fasting you break the power of your appetite and get beyond caffeine headaches. In several months do a five-day or ten-day fast. Ask the Lord for your strategy to enter into a fasting lifestyle. Also drink plenty of liquids. During a fast, toxins are being released from your body and you must flush them out with great quantities of liquids. Keep drinking liquids even when you are breaking an extended fast.

Breaking a fast is an important physical dimension of fasting. Break your fast carefully. After a fast of three days you can go back to normal eating immediately. Don't break your fast, however, on a big meal. For a fast that is over three or four days and extended fasts of twenty-one or forty days you must break your fast slowly. Increase your intake of food over several days or even several weeks depending on the length of your fast. Start by eating fruits. Then go to vegetables and soups without meat. Keep drinking plenty of liquids during the time you break your fast. The breaking of an extended fast is very important. If done wrongly it can cause physical problems and intense pain. Take your time getting back to your normal intake of food.

Pull back the reins of your appetite

Mentally you can develop a lifestyle of fasting by learning to control your appetite. There is a world of difference between your appetite and hunger. The cravings you wrestle with during a fast are not just from hunger but also from your appetite. Hunger is a physiological response of your body when you haven't eaten. Your appetite is a mental conditioning to food which creates a physical craving. For that reason you can have an appetite for ice-cream even when your stomach is full and your hunger satisfied.

During an extended fast you break the grip of your appetite because you are no longer responding to your mental signals. Control your cravings after a fast by saying "no" to certain foods or to too much food. If you don't put the brakes on your appetite after a fast it will come back with a vengeance. This makes it harder to enter the next fast. Discipline yourself after a fast. Control your thoughts and cravings for unhealthy food or too much food. This will keep your weight from taking wild swings and makes it easier to fast next time.

Watch out for the enemy

Spiritually you can help develop your fasting lifestyle by understanding the enemy's schemes to defeat you. Because fasting can unlock so many spiritual resources in the kingdom of God, Satan wants to keep you from using the fasting key.

Before a fast the enemy will try to bring disruptions and distractions to keep you from fasting or focusing in faith. During the fast the enemy may tempt you to come out of your fast before the time the Lord gave you. This is the same tactic he used against Jesus when He fasted in the wilderness (Matthew 4:3–4). If you break your fast too soon, don't get under a cloud of shame. That too is the enemy's weapon. He uses shame to keep you from fasting again. Instead of stalling out in shame, ask the Lord to forgive you. Then prepare yourself for the next fast. Remember that breaking a fast prematurely is not the unforgivable sin. Lighten up and ask the Lord to help you the next time. Fasting is not an all-or-nothing event. It is a developing lifestyle.

After a fast be on the lookout for two more weapons of the enemy. He can bring depression. Don't be tempted to think it was all for nothing. That is a scheme of Satan to steal the benefits of your fast. Stay in faith and consolidate the gains of your fast.

Avoid spiritual pride. Satan can tempt you into thinking you have done something wonderful. Don't use your fasting to prove your spiritual greatness. Everything is by God's grace. Fasting simply opens up your spirit to receive more grace. Fasting is not about the person fasting. It is all about Jesus.

Benefits of a fasting lifestyle

Many of the fasting experiences throughout this book are dramatic. They were chosen because dramatic illustrations can help us to view experiences as through a microscope – they are intended to magnify the results of fasting so that we see them in greater detail. Whether your experience with fasting is dramatic or quiet, however, the benefits are always rich. At times I have seen spectacular results through a fast and at other times I have known quiet workings of the Spirit. The joy of a fasting lifestyle is to see the unique way the Lord works through each fast.

I'll leave you with a portion of one more dramatic testimony. It comes from William Duma's first fast. This fast eventually led him into a lifestyle of fasting. On the last day of a twenty-one-day fast, Duma climbed a hill before dawn to worship the Lord. He covered himself with a coat because it was cold. Suddenly he felt warm and he thought the sun had risen. When he looked out from the coat he found he was in the center of dazzling light. It was the glory of God. William Duma describes the scene.

> "A curtain of shining gold, suspended in space slightly above the ground, completely encircled my dark figure . . . My hands no longer dark brown, were the color of golden honey . . . It was still dark out there against the pre-dawn blackness. Only my hilltop was covered by the golden circle of light . . . I thought, 'The Lord is here and I am not worthy.' "[1]

After this encounter God spoke specifically to William Duma about his life and ministry. He left the hilltop with the light of God's glory visibly shining from him. This experience began a lifestyle of fasting and a life of kingdom ministry.

Seek the Lord through a lifestyle of fasting. Whether you encounter His visible glory or not, you will encounter Him. The Lord Jesus Christ is the reason for your fast.

Note

1. Mary Garnett, *Take Your Glory Lord* (Kent: Sovereign World, 2000) pp. 26, 27